"In our postfeminist, hypersexualized culture, women are confused about what the Bible teaches about sexuality. *Sexual Sanity for Women* is an eminently practical small group resource that will minister to women who are addicted to pornography, struggle with same-sex attraction, feel guilty from a lifestyle of promiscuity, have been sexually abused, or just need to understand what Christianity has to say about sexuality. It deals with the issues frankly while pointing women to gospel truths in a compassionate way. A must-have resource for every women's ministry."

Melanie M. Cogdill, Managing Editor, Christian Research Journal

"In an age where gender and sexuality are central battlefronts of the Enemy, the church must be ready to respond. *Sexual Sanity for Women* has broken the 'louder silence' for women. Many resources are merely academic or self-help in nature. Yet, this curriculum is a thorough, rare, and vital tool that will equip ministry leaders, counselors, and the church to bring hope and help to the sexually broken. Its comprehensive perspective effectively facilitates personal and corporate reflection while remaining Christ-centered, ultimately unpacking how the gospel speaks to gender and sexuality."

Heather Evans, *LCSW*, Counselor in private practice, Coopersburg, PA and cofounder of The Valley Against Sex Trafficking (VAST) Coalition

"Sexual Sanity for Women: Healing from Sexual and Relational Brokenness is way overdue. A generation of iKids has known sexuality from the perspective of technology and the internet. We need solid resources to help us teach those entering our church settings with heart-wrenching stories how to push the 'reset button' on their sexuality. Ellen Dykas has edited a creatively useful handbook for the church and counselors working with any woman who needs to retrain her heart to think about sexuality as a gift from God. This is a solid resource to use with teens, college women, or new believers. Harvest USA has hit the nail on the head yet again."

Dr. Penny Nelson Freeman, *LPC*, The Counseling Center at Chelten

"Ellen Dykas and the staff of Harvest USA have written a compassionate, insightful, and practical book that is faithful to God's Word in addressing the relational and sexual brokenness unique to women. This book speaks with truth and love to the issues that women in our churches are facing. The gospel of Jesus Christ applied in this way will bring hope and freedom to many."

Ron Lutz, Pastor, New Life Presbyterian Church, Dresher, PA

SEXUAL SANITY
FOR WOMEN
HEALING FROM SEXUAL
AND RELATIONAL BROKENNESS

Harvest USA

Ellen Dykas, Editor

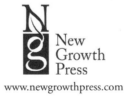

New
Growth
Press

www.newgrowthpress.com

New Growth Press, Greensboro, NC 27404
Copyright ©2012 by Harvest USA.

Sexual Sanity for Women: Healing from Sexual and Relational Brokenness is based on portions of *DIG: Daughters in Grace*, an unpublished women's curriculum developed by Sarah Lipp for Harvest USA, copyright © 2008 by Harvest USA.

Cover Design: Faceout Studios, Tim Green
Interior Design and Typesetting: Lisa Parnell, lparnell.com

ISBN 978-1-938267-00-0

Printed in Canada

19 18 17 16 15 14 13 12   1 2 3 4 5

CONTENTS

Appendices

INTRODUCTION

Welcome! The women's ministry of Harvest USA exists to minister the gospel of grace to women who are struggling with relational and sexual brokenness. We hope this study, *Sexual Sanity for Women: Healing from Sexual and Relational Brokenness,* will provide a tool that can be used in churches, communities, and life-on-life relationships. Our desire is that women would be equipped and encouraged by the gospel of Jesus Christ, so they love him and grow in freedom from the sin and pain of relational and sexual brokenness.

What does it mean to be relationally and/or sexually broken? The Bible clearly states that all have sinned and fallen short of the glory of God (Romans 3:23). The impact of sin has had a devastating effect on all of creation. One aspect of this utter ruin is that nothing functions in the way our Creator originally intended. Our world is broken. Relational and sexual brokenness thus refers to the sin struggles and temptations that women and men battle against while they live on this earth. Relationships become a prime ground for our idols to be nurtured and developed, as we seek people to be what only Christ can be. Sex becomes a way to medicate the pain within our hearts—or to feel anything at all. Our gender and sexual identity become confused, blurred, and even frightening. All things may have been created through Jesus and for Jesus (Colossians 1:16), but no one experiences life entirely according to his good design. Our lives are broken—but the gospel of healing, restoration, and forgiveness *has broken into our brokenness!*

Women are sexual beings just as much as men are. However, they often experience an even "louder silence" regarding their sexual sin and temptation. The Christian community has taken slow steps in recent years to address issues of sexuality, including addictions of a sexual nature. However, the opportunities for women to have the gospel specifically applied to their areas of relational

1

and sexual brokenness have been few and far between. It's our hope that *Sexual Sanity for Women* will provide opportunities for women to gather together and receive encouragement and teaching that will help them to, "lay aside every weight, and sin which clings so closely, and let [them] run with endurance the race that is set before [them], looking to Jesus, the founder and perfecter of our faith, who for the joy that was set before him endured the cross, despising the shame, and is seated at the right hand of the throne of God" (Hebrews 12:1–2).

A few thoughts as you begin to work through this study. Although an individual could journey through it herself, this material is meant to be used in a group setting. There is power in people coming together to walk in the light with one another, confessing weakness and sin, praying for one other, and urging each other on in the calling to put on the Lord Jesus Christ and to make no provision for fleshly desires (Romans 13:14). This process of throwing off sinful patterns of life is just that—*a process!* This material will assist women to begin that process of freedom and change, and gives strugglers a place *to start* in addressing these deeply held and usually carefully guarded issues.

Many women who wrestle with their sexuality in sinful ways—including promiscuity, pornography, fantasy life, masturbation, and homosexuality—have other heart struggles as well. The Bible is clear that we all live out of our hearts, and yet our hearts have been impacted by living in a sinful world, where people sin against one another in traumatic ways. This study is not meant to provide in-depth counseling for the pain brought on by trauma and abuse. Professional counseling and/or pastoral counseling by wise, mature Christians is highly recommended as part of this process of opening up one's personal history and struggles. Ultimately, healing and change is the work of our Savior Jesus Christ, who came to heal the brokenhearted and to set the captive free—including female captives and daughters of God who are brokenhearted!

For groups, here are several guidelines that each woman should commit to:

- Faithful attendance and commitment, for the duration of the group (twenty sessions)
- Wisdom in sharing of struggles and sin patterns. This means sharing enough to be known, but not details that will leave graphic images in the minds of other women.

- Engaging the homework and reflective questions/readings, with a commitment to learn and grow
- Seeking to be a trustworthy woman by not sharing anything outside the group, except for her own personal stories of growth
- Keeping a private prayer and processing journal of what you are learning is also encouraged, but not required!

Talk to your group leader if you have questions or concerns regarding these important guidelines.

One final note about the process of change: Remember, change *is* a process and, generally, it's experienced over time. It may involve a person going back briefly to familiar sin, or learning to accept that certain temptations may remain while one lives out her earthly life. In other words, the very definition of what change *is* often changes in a women's life. Hence, earlier expectations of what one hoped for may not be met—or may be exceeded. Either way, the Lord is faithful to transform our lives as we surrender to him, trusting in the work of the Holy Spirit to conform us more and more into women of whom it could be said, "*She lived a life of following Christ, and his presence was increasingly evident in her life!*" May God grant you wisdom, hope, and grace as you go through this material. Our prayer is that much glory will come to King Jesus as women are set free to love, serve, and worship him.

SESSION 1
GETTING STARTED

KEY CONCEPT: In order to experience freedom from sinful relationships, sexual patterns, and desires, we need to understand that these behaviors are expressions of a sinful heart that has been influenced by a sinful world. Change begins as we address the deeper heart issues in our lives, through the truth and grace of God's Word.

SESSION 1—GETTING STARTED

Welcome (20 minutes)

Ask the women to read the following passage to themselves. Then discuss the questions that follow:

Today's culture shouts out messages promising ultimate satisfaction in this life—often through relationships and sexual experiences. The Bible teaches that God created relationships and sexual intimacy as gifts for people to enjoy, but within his ordained context. God's good design for sexuality is for both men and women!

However women, like men, wrestle with sexual brokenness through the pursuit of what God calls "broken cisterns" (see Jeremiah 2:13)—sources of life, security, and value that we look for in this world rather than in its Creator. Sexual and relational sin are examples of broken cisterns that women run to and have sought to find soul satisfaction in, rather than finding true life in God. *Sexual Sanity for Women* is for women seeking to grow in loving and obeying Jesus and to be increasingly free from sinful sexual and relational patterns. The sessions to come will guide women into a deeper understanding of God's good design for sexuality, how and why women struggle with sexual brokenness, and how the grace and truth of Jesus Christ can be applied to these struggles.

1. What one or two hopes or goals do you have for yourself, as you participate in this group and work through this study?

2. What are you most excited and/or fearful about, as you seek change regarding your relational patterns, sexual behaviors, and desires?

Exploring the Key Issue (60 minutes)

Read the Key Concept, and then discuss the questions that follow:

Key Concept: In order to experience freedom from sinful relationships, sexual patterns, and desires, we need to understand that these behaviors are expressions of a sinful heart that has been influenced by a sinful world. Change begins as we address the deeper heart issues in our lives through the truth and grace of God's Word.

3. What have you understood to be the causes of your specific sin struggles?

4. What is your understanding about what the Bible teaches about our struggles?

5. Have you ever felt drawn into a relationship or behavior to the point that you've felt you couldn't stop yourself? What did that feel like? Why do you think it happened?

destructive

fear
all-consuming - obsessed
weak
guilt + shame pwords
temporary high, then the low

Read the following passage, and then discuss the questions that follow:

Sexual addictions among women are rarely talked about. Women strugglers often feel loaded down with a heavy sense of shame. They feel they are somehow "extra-abnormal" because sexual sin is typically addressed only as a man's problem. When we consider female homosexuality and same-sex attraction, there is confusion in the way it is discussed and understood. We hear many explanations about why individuals are attracted to the same gender. There has been a major push in the media to say that homosexuality is something that's inborn and unchangeable ("I was born this way"). Even within many faith communities, there has been growing acceptance of homosexuality as a God-blessed identity ("I'm a gay Christian").

How does a biblical view inform not only the question, "Is being gay OK?", but what homosexuality *is*? And does the Bible really address seemingly "private" sexual activities such as viewing and reading pornography or masturbation? And if I truly love and am committed to someone, what's the big deal in expressing myself sexually with that person outside marriage? Finally, does God really have helpful advice about addictions in our lives, especially those of a sexual or emotional nature?

We'll explore these hard but important questions in the sessions to come. What we'll learn will give us hope and confidence that God's Word *does* speak into all these sensitive areas. Through the person of Jesus, God has given us more than a set of rules to follow or a series of steps to complete. He loves us and is actually after so much more than behavioral change. He is able to transform our hearts and minds and grow us into Christlike women!

The gospel of Jesus Christ speaks to every struggler—woman or man, younger or older. And whether the sinful pattern takes the shape of sexual promiscuity (with men, women, or both), homosexuality, emotionally enmeshed dependencies, or habitual sexual patterns (such as masturbation, pornography, or an obsessive fantasy life), God's Word has hope for real change. This study will explore how these patterns develop and how, through faith in Jesus Christ and obedience to the truths of the gospel, new Christlike patterns can grow and flourish in the life of any woman.

6. What thoughts or feelings do you have in response to the above?

7. Consider the quote: "Through the person of Jesus, God has given us more than a set of rules to follow, or a series of steps to complete. He loves us and is actually after so much more than behavioral change. He is able to transform our hearts and minds, and grow us into Christlike women!" As you think about your own sexual and relational struggles, does this idea seem hopeful, scary, overwhelming, encouraging, or something else? Explain.

God is about who we are, not what I'm doing.

8. Another way of defining addiction is a habitual (but changeable) pattern of behaving, thinking, and relating. Do you agree? Why or why not?

A pattern does not need to define who we are - it is not our identity.

9. Is it uncomfortable for you to discuss your sexual and relational struggles in the context of what God and the Bible say? Again, why or why not?

pleasure pathways in brain + needs more - continues to escalate.

Making It Personal (15 minutes)

Read the following passage together:

Jesus consistently describes behavior as coming out of the heart of a person. He puts it this way, "The tree is known by its fruit" (Matthew 12:33; Luke 6:43–45). He also says that it's not what we put into our mouths that corrupt us, but what comes out of our mouths (our words) that corrupt us. He says the mouth speaks from out of the heart (Matthew 12:34). What Jesus seems to be saying is that the inner issues are what really drive us, and what we say or do reveals our hearts. Jesus consistently focuses on what's inside a person, not just on outward manifestations of behavior. He compared the behavior of religious leaders to cups that were clean on the outside but dirty on the inside (Matthew 23:25).

Jesus was very compassionate to individuals struggling with sexual sin. He showed great love and compassion to *women who are sexual strugglers* (Luke 7:36–48; John 4:7–26; and 8:1–11). If you were to encounter Jesus today, you could have confidence that he would not condemn you but would show you love and mercy. You could also be confident to know that he would not focus exclusively on your outward behaviors and sins, but rather on the deeper motivational issues that arise from the core of who you are in your heart.

Beginning to deal with your sexual behaviors, relational struggles and emotional attractions can be very scary and difficult. The purpose of this group is to provide a setting where you can deal with some painful and troubling issues within a caring and supportive group setting.

This study will guide you through a model for understanding behavior called the Tree Model. It's based on what Jesus said about being able to tell a tree by its fruit. This model will become critical to your understanding of why you do what you do. Remember, God is seeking much more than outward change through transformed behaviors! He is seeking heart change—which means that the deeper, inner issues in your life will be addressed and then "re-dressed" with the grace and truth of Jesus. True change and healing is possible, as we set our focus on Jesus Christ who has come to heal the brokenhearted and set the captives free!

On Your Own (5 minutes)

1. Read 2 Corinthians 1:3–4. God is a gracious Father and is full of comfort. In what ways do you need to be comforted, as you consider the pain your sin has caused you and others?

2. Read Luke 6:43–45. Reflect on how your specific sin struggles are the fruit of deeper issues within your heart.

SESSION 2
OUT OF THE HEART: THE TREE MODEL

KEY CONCEPT: Scripture often compares people to trees—and from the fruit it bears, we can tell what kind of tree it is. The Harvest USA Tree Model is a way to understand how our sin patterns develop as a result of our sinful hearts being impacted by a variety of influences, and how through Jesus Christ, our hearts (our *real* problem) can be transformed more and more into his likeness.

SESSION 2—OUT OF THE HEART: THE TREE MODEL

Review and Reflect (15 minutes)

Review last week's Key Concept, and then discuss the questions that follow:

Last Week's Key Concept: To experience freedom from sinful sexual and relational patterns, we need to understand that these behaviors are expressions of a sinful heart that has been influenced by living in a sinful world. Change begins as we address the deeper heart issues in our lives through the truth, grace, and wisdom of God's Word.

1. What insights have you had over the past week, as you reflected on the idea that our sexual behaviors are the fruit of our hearts?

2. Share insights from 2 Corinthians 1:3–4. How do these verses speak to you in your desire to become more like Christ and to be free from sexual sins?

Exploring the Key Issue (60 minutes)

Key Concept: Scripture often compares people to trees—and from the fruit it bears, we can tell what kind of tree it is. The Harvest USA Tree Model is a way to understand how our sin patterns develop as a result of our sinful hearts being impacted by a variety of influences, and how through Jesus Christ, our hearts (our *real* problem) can be transformed more and more into his likeness.

Jesus tells us in Luke 6:45 that our behaviors are not merely the result of something acting upon us from the outside (other people, pain, being sinned against, circumstances, etc.), but arise out of the heart. The Tree Model explains how the connection between our behaviors and our hearts can be understood. A tree is made of several parts—fruit, seed, roots, shoots, and the soil in which the seed is planted, and begins to grow. This session will give an overview for you to begin to interact with these concepts; the next several sessions will explore these components in more detail.

Review the Tree Model, and the descriptions that follow, as a group. After reading each description, take two to three minutes to quietly reflect and

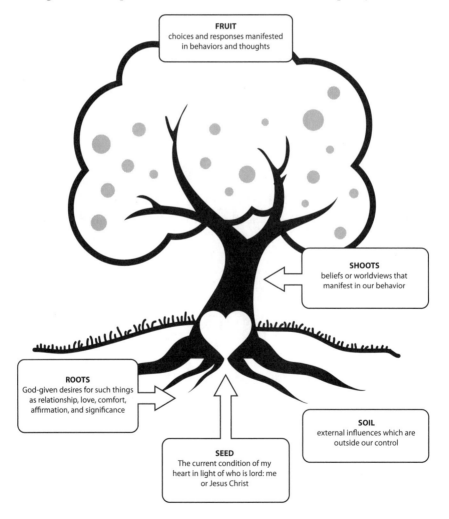

FRUIT
choices and responses manifested in behaviors and thoughts

SHOOTS
beliefs or worldviews that manifest in our behavior

ROOTS
God-given desires for such things as relationship, love, comfort, affirmation, and significance

SOIL
external influences which are outside our control

SEED
The current condition of my heart in light of who is lord: me or Jesus Christ

write your answer to the question that follows. Do this for all five descriptions (questions 3–7).

Fruit—The fruit on our tree represents our behavior or present struggles. These are the reasons we ask others for help, or go see a counselor. Among these struggles are our thoughts, behaviors, and relational patterns. Examples include envy, anger, anxiety, overeating, gossip, homosexual behavior, sexual fantasies, looking at pornography, sexual promiscuity, and masturbation. However, fruit can also be holy and of the Spirit, as Galatians 5:22–23 teaches us.

3. What fruit in your life do you want to see changed? Share as much as you're willing.

Seed—The seed represents our heart, or soul, which is the spiritual center of each person. It's what makes each of us unique as a woman created by God. It's the seat of our will. It is "us." Yet the Bible teaches us that we all have a big problem: We're sinners! "If we say we have no sin, we deceive ourselves, and the truth is not in us" (1 John 1:8). Our sinful heart/seed makes self the center as we experience life and relationships in this world. We are born sinners, completely in need of Jesus Christ to give us a new heart. Jesus Christ, through his death and resurrection, has made it possible for anyone who comes to him for forgiveness of sin to be made a new creation through a new heart that desires new—and better—fruit. While we live on this earth we'll continue to battle against temptation and won't live a sin-free life, but over time we will grow in Christlikeness as we turn from self toward our Savior. The Bible calls this process *repentance*. It is key that we understand this, in order to grow into increasing freedom over life-dominating sin patterns, whether they're are sexual, relational, or other.

4. Have you confessed your sin to God and received his forgiveness? First John 1:9 promises that if we confess our sins to God, he is faithful and just to forgive us of all sin, and to cleanse us of everything that is not right in our

lives. Write a few thoughts about your experience of God's forgiveness, as you understand it right now.

Roots—Roots refer to God-given desires for relationship, intimacy, and significance which, due to our sinful nature, are bent toward seeking satisfaction in selfish, me-oriented ways. The Bible calls this pursuit of self "idolatry." Idolatry originates from a selfish sinful heart that craves satisfaction in ways outside of God's design. This is a woman, desiring to be loved and cherished, lusting for sexual attention from a man because it makes her feel loved. This is a woman enmeshed emotionally and sexually with another woman because it feels comforting and secure to be someone's #1. This is a woman who watches porn and escapes to a fantasy world of her own making because it's a world of relationships in which she feels no pain and always gets what she wants. Common desires, when expressed from a self-serving heart, quickly grow into selfish demands, thus bearing the fruit of sexual and relational sin.

5. What desires can you identify in yourself that seem to exert the most control over you and that have fueled your patterns of sinful relationships and sexual behavior? (Desires for comfort, love, intimacy, control, to feel significant, to not feel pain, bodily pleasure, etc.)

Soil—The soil represents influences upon our lives that shape us, influence us, and encourage us toward certain patterns for dealing with life. Although they can be positive or negative, hurtful or praiseworthy, we ultimately cannot blame them for where and who we are today. We've already seen how our behaviors are born out of our hearts. However, living in a broken world of sin—in which we are sinned against and experience pain, suffering, joy and blessing, healthy and unhealthy relationships, etc.—*does* impact us. Various soil influences include:

- Temperament and emotional makeup
- The voice and values of culture, peers, and society
- Family dynamics
- Gender
- Body type
- Talents and personal strengths/gifts
- Abuse (physical, sexual, emotional)
- Trauma through death, abandonment, painful losses, etc.
- Physiology and other biological factors
- Spiritual warfare (the kingdom of darkness which opposes God and his purposes in our lives)

6. What aspects of soil jump off the page immediately as ones you can recognize as having a strong influence in your life? Why those?

Shoots—The shoots of the tree are the conclusions or worldviews we've developed over the years. Think of the shoots as the lenses through which we view and interpret our world—how we believe "life works." Our interpretations, however, are always tainted by self, thus proving our lifelong need for transformed minds to think according to God's truth. We live, relate, respond, and behave out of our faulty understandings of God, men, women, relationships, sex, gender, etc. For example: "I must speak only nice things so that others like me"; "I'm worthless and undesirable"; "All men want one thing from women"; "Emotional pain is death to me, so I need to avoid any discomfort and pursue only what feels good"; "I'm valued and secure if others need me"; "People are untrustworthy, so it's best to just stay to myself and let no one really know me"; "God didn't protect me, so God doesn't love me"; "Being a woman is power"; "Being female is worthless." Although these convictions fuel our choices, they often develop unconsciously and thus are not on our mental radar screen most of the time. When we are unaware of the inner beliefs which drive our behavior, it's challenging to understand why we do what we do—the fruit being born out of our hearts.

7. Think of the primary focus of your sin struggles: a mental fantasy world and/or pornography, men, women, both, sex with yourself. What do you crave from this experience, type of person, or type of relationship? What are you seeking to avoid and escape through it?

lonely, not chosen   a quick high - but tends to bring even lower.
false sense of intimacy.

Discuss the following questions as a group:

8. When we consider a person as a "tree" it may seem overwhelming to put it all together! Let's take the example of a woman who comes to you for help in her Christian life and:

- Identifies herself as a gay woman
- Desires to love and obey Jesus
- Knows that she can't have both a homosexual lifestyle and a life of obedience to God
- Desires having a person with whom she can share life
- Believes that men are unsafe, as most of her experiences with men have led to her being taken advantage of and misused sexually
- Is having a difficult time cutting off contact with her recent girlfriend, even though she knows she must take this step of obedience. They continue to keep tabs on each other through social media and texting, and occasionally see each other when mutual friends get together.

What do you think are the first steps to take to help her? Why?

9. Read these passages together, and discuss how they correspond to the individual components of the Tree Model:

- Mark 12:28–31
- Colossians 3:1–3
- 2 Corinthians 5:14–17
- Romans 12:1–2
- Isaiah 61:1–3

Making It Personal (10 minutes)

For some people, it's a major shift in thinking to begin focusing on deeper issues rather than surface behaviors. We often want to feel better or get fixed so badly that we simply want the behaviors to stop. We want a program that will do a quick fix or provide a series of steps that will change our behaviors. In most cases a programmatic approach to changing behavior fails because behaviors are merely symptoms of a deeper problem: Our hearts are sinful and in need of change. Our desires need to be understood as our servants and not our masters. We let them serve us in leading us to God in a variety of ways—asking for help or blessing, crying out for comfort or encouragement, giving thanks, praising him, etc. Our thought lives need radical transformation in order to be aligned with God's truth and ways.

The gospel of Jesus Christ is the good news not only that he *said* he came to save, change, and heal us, but that he's *able* to do this! The next several sessions will further explore the inner dynamics of your heart and how life in this world has impacted and shaped your thoughts. It may be very painful and frustrating. It may seem like you're getting nowhere and that your struggles only intensify. Don't give up. Healing and change is a process. A broken bone does not heal overnight—neither does a spiritually broken heart!

On Your Own (5 minutes)

1. Review the scriptures in Question 9, and journal about how they encourage and help you to have your heart set on Jesus more than on your struggles.

2. Fill in the "My Tree" sheet, and come next week prepared to share two or three details from each component. Review the guidelines on sharing in a group context, on p. 2 of the Introduction.

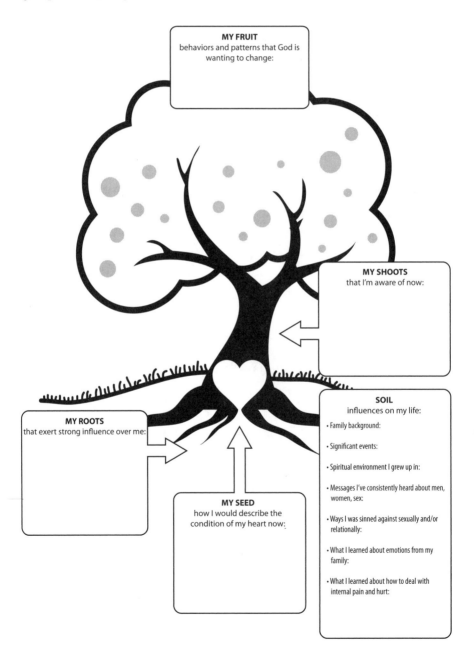

MY FRUIT
behaviors and patterns that God is wanting to change:

MY SHOOTS
that I'm aware of now:

MY ROOTS
that exert strong influence over me:

SOIL
influences on my life:

• Family background:

• Significant events:

• Spiritual environment I grew up in:

• Messages I've consistently heard about men, women, sex:

• Ways I was sinned against sexually and/or relationally:

• What I learned about emotions from my family:

• What I learned about how to deal with internal pain and hurt:

MY SEED
how I would describe the condition of my heart now:

SESSION 3
APPLYING THE TREE TO *ME*

KEY CONCEPT: People are much more alike than they are different. We all need God's grace, wisdom, and love as we live life in this world. Regardless of what patterns of struggle and sin (fruit) we each have battled against, the source is the same—our wayward hearts. Regardless of how we have suffered and been sinned against, our need is the same—the healing grace of Jesus Christ. As we get to know each other through the details of our experiences, we'll grow in being wise helpers to others as we're enabled to apply specific truths of God's grace, to specific pain, sins, and questions.

SESSION 3—APPLYING THE TREE TO *ME*

Review and Reflect (15 minutes)

Open your session in prayer. Review last week's Key Concept, and then discuss the questions that follow:

Last Week's Key Concept: Scripture often compares people to a tree, explaining that we can tell by the fruit born from a tree what kind of tree it is! *The Harvest USA Tree Model* is a way to understand (a) how our sin patterns develop as a result of our sinful hearts being impacted by a variety of influences and (b) how through Jesus Christ our hearts can be transformed more and more into his likeness.

1. What insights did you gain as you reviewed the Tree Model? What questions, if any, do you have about it?

2. What encouragement or insights did you get out of the Scripture passages you reviewed? What questions arose from your readings?

Exploring the Key Issue (60 minutes)

Read the following together, then discuss the questions that follow:

Key Concept: People are much more alike than they are different. We all need God's grace, wisdom, and love as we live life in this world. Regardless of what patterns of struggle and sin (fruit) we each have battled against, the source is the same—our wayward hearts. Regardless of how we have suffered and been sinned against, our need is the same—the healing grace of Jesus Christ. As we get to know each other through the details of our experiences, we'll grow in being wise helpers to others as we're enabled to apply specific truths of God's grace to specific pain, sins, and questions.

This week we'll "do" the Key Concept, by sharing key points that came to light as we mapped our lives onto the Tree Model. Scripture teaches that growth in grace and Christlikeness happens as we pursue growth *together*. As we "walk in the light" (1 John 1:7), God guides us to be people who have an openness with him about our struggles (confession and receiving forgiveness), as well as with each other about our struggles (being known). It's been well said that the power of secret sin is in the secret. This session will give each woman an opportunity to be known through sharing a few specifics regarding:

- Your fruit: What are the specific sexual and/or relational sin patterns you struggle with?
- Your soil: At this point in your life, what shaping influences or experiences are you aware of? What kind of impact have they had upon you?
- Your roots: What desires seem to easily hijack your heart and lean you toward living selfishly?
- Your shoots: What are some of the interpretations or worldviews you're aware of that fuel your behavior and attitudes?
- Your seed: How would you describe your desire and commitment to grow in loving God and surrendering your life to him?

Take time now to share your reflections from the past week together, and from your work on the Tree Model on p. 20. Remember: We're only beginning this journey! Some women may have insight into all of the above; others may struggle to think of anything beyond the obvious sinful fruit in her life. This is just a start, so that each person can share about her past history and begin to get to know other women in the group.

3. What similar themes did you notice as you listened to the things shared from the group, including your own insights? How surprised were you to discover this? Explain.

Making It Personal (10 minutes)

Jesus said:

> "The Spirit of the Lord is upon me, because he has anointed me to proclaim good news to the poor. He has sent me to proclaim liberty to the captives and recovering of sight to the blind, to set at liberty those who are oppressed, to proclaim the year of the Lord's favor." (Luke 4:18–19)

Jesus offers these ministries to each person who will come to him in humility and ask for help. As we apply the Tree Model to our lives, we not only grow in understanding how and why we've been captive to sin, blind to God's truth, and living under spiritual oppression—we grow in knowing *him*! Jesus was anointed and sent for these very reasons. That's good news for each of us, regardless of what our sexual sin has been. God alone has the power and the loving grace to change our hearts and grow us into women who resemble a fruitful, Christ-like tree!

On Your Own (5 minutes)

1. Read 1 John 1:5–10; James 5:16; and Proverbs 28:13. Reflect on what these passages teach about walking in the light with other people in regard to our sin struggles. What are the benefits of being committed to journeying openly with others and not hiding from them? Write them down here.

2. Our next session is a brief overview of God's design for sexuality, for both the married and unmarried. If we want to grow as women who are increasingly Christlike in how we express our sexuality, we need to understand what God says. Read the article "God's Design for Sexuality" in Appendix A (p. 168), and answer these questions:

    a.   What stood out to you from this article? How were you encouraged?

    b.   Do you disagree with anything in the article? What, and why?

    c.   God's design for sexuality is radically different from our culture's, and even from what many professing Christians actually live out. Why do you think so many Christians struggle to obey God in their sexual lives?

SESSION 4
THE FRUIT: GODLY SEXUALITY

KEY CONCEPT: How we express ourselves as sexual beings is one of the fruits of our hearts—expressing either submission to Christ or slavery to self. God's design for sex and sexuality has a good, Christ-honoring expression for both the married and unmarried. He gives marriage as a gift and provides the context for sexual expression. God also gives singleness as a gift and provides the context for Christ-enabled fasting from sexual expression. Godly sexuality, for both the married and unmarried, is meant to be a signpost to Christ and a means by which we love God and others.

SESSION 4—THE FRUIT: GODLY SEXUALITY

Review and Reflect (15 minutes)

Open your session in prayer. Review last week's Key Concept, and then discuss the questions that follow:

Last Week's Key Concept: People are much more alike than they are different. We all need God's grace, wisdom, and love as we live life in this world. Regardless of what patterns of struggle and sin (fruit) we each have battled against, the source is the same—our wayward hearts. Regardless of how we have suffered and been sinned against, our need is the same—the healing grace of Jesus Christ. As we get to know each other through the details of our experiences, we'll grow in being wise helpers to others as we're enabled to apply specific truths of God's grace to specific pain, sins, and questions.

1. What did you discover from reading 1 John 1:5–10; James 5:16; and Proverbs 28:13, especially in terms of the benefits of walking in the light with others?

2. What are the risks of confessing your sins and weaknesses (James 5:16) to others?

Exploring the Key Issue (60 minutes)

Read this week's Key Concept:

Key Concept: How we express ourselves as sexual beings is one of the fruits of our hearts, expressing either submission to Christ or slavery to self. God's design for sex and sexuality has a good, Christ-honoring expression for both the married and unmarried. He gives marriage as a gift and provides the context for sexual expression. God also gives singleness as a gift and provides the context for Christ-enabled fasting from sexual expression. Godly sexuality, for both the married and unmarried, is meant to be a signpost to Christ and a means by which we love God and others.

Discuss last week's reading, "God's Design for Sexuality" (found in Appendix A on p. 168), using the following questions:

3. What stood out to you from this article? How were you encouraged? Were you surprised by anything?

4. Do you disagree with any of the points in the article regarding why God has designed sexual expression to be contained within the marriage relationship, which he defines as one man with one woman for life? If so, why?

5. Discuss the main points for both godly married and unmarried sexuality and share what are the most challenging aspects for you to accept. How does it make a difference to know that God is Creator and Designer, as you seek to live a godly sexual life?

6. God's design for sexuality is radically different from the voice of our culture and even from what many professing Christians are actually living out. Why do you think so many Christians struggle to obey God in their sexual lives?

Making It Personal (10 minutes)

The article "God's Design for Sexuality" gives an overview of the "what and why" of what the Bible teaches, not only regarding sinful sexual activity but what it means to express our sexuality in God-honoring ways. Oftentimes God is left out of discussions of sex— which is unwise since he's the Creator! God is also the Father of compassion (2 Corinthians 1:3–4) who comforts us as we struggle to live out sexual holiness. He provides and protects us as his children, who are utterly in need of him in order to live obedient sexual lives.

Another quality of our God is that he is Lord; we belong to him and not to ourselves. The world screams autonomy and self-ownership through messages such as, "Don't tell me what I can or can't do with my body!" and "Get your religious rules out of my sex life!" Yet our loving Father and wise Creator is also the one we are called to serve. Our service to him includes surrender and obedience in stewarding our bodies and our sexuality.

We are deeply loved, and we are lovingly created and owned by God. Living out a godly sexuality, whether single or married, will call us not only to wisely align our hearts with what he tells us to obey, but to know and love him. He is for us, not against us. His commands are for our flourishing and for his glory!

On Your Own (5 minutes)

Sessions 5 and 6 will unpack why ungodly fruit of a sexual nature is sinful. When our desires and the messages we've heard from the world have been the loudest voices in our hearts and minds, God's design can seem anything but fair or doable. Take time this week to reflect on these Bible passages that describe God, who is the Creator of sexuality and the Designer of how we're intended to experience it. Pray and ask him to reveal himself to you, to give you a humble and teachable heart, and to encourage you as you seek to walk forward in being a woman conformed to the image of Jesus.

Reflect upon these passages:

- Psalm 23 (This may be a familiar passage to you. Read it with fresh eyes, as you seek to learn how God is a shepherd to you in your sexual temptations and desires.)
- Colossians 1:1–23 (specifically Paul's prayer in verses 9–12)

SESSION 5
THE FRUIT: UNDERSTANDING FEMALE SEXUAL SIN

KEY CONCEPT: In contrast to God's design for sex, sexual sin is the fruit of a self-ruled and idolatrous heart. Sexual activity outside marriage (with women or men)—with self (masturbation), with someone else's spouse, sexual fantasy, and the viewing and reading of pornography—are ways women seek sexual pleasure and emotional comfort outside God's wise boundaries. These behaviors are the fruit of a heart living against God's created design for sexual expression.

SESSION 5—THE FRUIT: UNDERSTANDING FEMALE SEXUAL SIN

Review and Reflect (15 minutes)

Open your session in prayer. Review last week's Key Concept, and then discuss the questions that follow:

Last Week's Key Concept: How we express ourselves as sexual beings is one of the fruits of our hearts—expressing either submission to Christ or slavery to self. God's design for sex and sexuality has a good, Christ-honoring expression for both the married and unmarried. He gives marriage as a gift and provides the context for sexual expression. God also gives singleness as a gift and provides the context for Christ-enabled fasting from sexual expression. Godly sexuality, for both the married and unmarried, is meant to be a signpost to Christ and a means by which we love God and others.

1. How did your reading of Psalm 23 impact you, as you considered what it says about the Lord as our Shepherd and how our sexual sin is among our struggles as his sheep?

2. How can you apply Paul's prayer in Colossians 1:9–12 to your desire to grow as a woman who walks in a manner worthy of God and bears fruit that pleases him? Be specific.

Exploring the Key Issue (60 minutes)

Read this week's Key Concept:

Key Concept: In contrast to God's design for sex, sexual sin is the fruit of a self-ruled and idolatrous heart. Sexual activity outside marriage (with women or men)—with self (masturbation), with someone else's spouse, sexual fantasy, and the viewing and reading of pornography—are ways women seek sexual pleasure and emotional comfort outside God's wise boundaries. These behaviors are the fruit of a heart living against God's created design for sexual expression.

Read the following passage silently, and then discuss the questions that follow.

All things have been created by Jesus and for Jesus (Colossians 1:16), and the Bible says that we can do all things through Christ who strengthens us (Philippians 4:13). If these things are true, then why do we struggle so much to live godly lives? Why is the battle to be faithful and obedient to Christ as sexual beings so hard? And why is it that sexual and relational sins seem so ingrained in us, provoking a deep sense of shame, sadness, or of being overcome? Is sexual sin a worse sin, in a category of its own?

For all the categories of sin that people have comprised, and the creative ways we describe "our issues," God's Word is crisp and clear in its diagnosis of any sin. God's people, the Israelites, had been involved in all the categories and possible issues that we struggle with—anger, fear, sexual perversion, hatred, unbelief, gossip, jealousy, murder, pride, and envy, to name just a few. God sums their sin up this way:

> "Has a nation changed its gods,
>   even though they are no gods?
> But my people have changed their glory
>   for that which does not profit.
> Be appalled, O heavens, at this;
>   be shocked, be utterly desolate,
> declares the LORD,
> for my people have committed two evils:
> they have forsaken me,
>   the fountain of living waters,
> and hewed out cisterns for themselves,
>   broken cisterns that can hold no water." (Jeremiah 2:11–13)

When all is said and done, God summarizes the sin of his people with two truths:

    a.   They turned *away* from him, the source of true life (living water).

    b.   They chose to dig out and turn *toward* their own cisterns (or wells), in a selfish search for what they thought was "living water."

This turning away from God to other things for life and satisfaction is what the Bible calls idolatry. Sexual sin is one of the ways that women turn away from God and try to make life work on their own terms. Later sessions will explore why we do this. For now, consider the clarity that God brings to our sin! The more specific we can be in naming it, the more specifically we'll be able to turn from it and receive the Lord's forgiveness and cleansing from the pollution it's brought into our lives (1 John 1:9–10).

3. What messages have you heard from Christians about sexual sin? Avoid names, but be specific about the messages themselves. How have those messages made you feel?

4. How have you been aware of turning *from* God, and seeking your own "fountain of living water" through your sexual sin?

5. How do you think Jesus dealt with women who were sexual sinners? Do you think he ever implied that sexual sin was worse than others or that women who sinned sexually were worse off than men? Explain.

Read the section below, and then discuss the questions that follow:

The New Testament is harmonious with the Old Testament's teaching concerning sin—it is to be turned away from as we turn to God (repentance). First Thessalonians 1:9 says, "For they themselves report concerning us the kind of reception we had among you, and how you turned to God from idols to serve the living and true God." The Thessalonians turned *from* their idols and sin because they were committed to turning to God.

In his letter to the Galatians, Paul shared more insights about the change process of turning from sin, including sins of a sexual nature. While not specifically listed, sins such as viewing or reading pornography, masturbation, casual sex, and engaging in a sexual fantasy life would all be included under sexual immorality. Paul encouraged followers of Jesus with these words:

> For you were called to freedom, brothers. Only do not use your freedom as an opportunity for the flesh, but through love serve one another. For the whole law is fulfilled in one word: "You shall love your neighbor as yourself." But if you bite and devour one another, watch out that you are not consumed by one another.
>
> But I say, walk by the Spirit, and you will not gratify the desires of the flesh. For the desires of the flesh are against the Spirit, and the desires of the Spirit are against the flesh, for these are opposed to each other, to keep you from doing the things you want to do. But if you are led by the Spirit, you are not under the law. Now the works of the flesh are evident: sexual immorality, impurity, sensuality, idolatry, sorcery, enmity, strife, jealousy, fits of anger, rivalries, dissensions, divisions, envy, drunkenness, orgies, and things

like these. I warn you, as I warned you before, that those who do such things will not inherit the kingdom of God. But the fruit of the Spirit is love, joy, peace, patience, kindness, goodness, faithfulness, gentleness, self-control; against such things there is no law. And those who belong to Christ Jesus have crucified the flesh with its passions and desires.

If we live by the Spirit, let us also keep in step with the Spirit. Let us not become conceited, provoking one another, envying one another. (Galatians 5:13–26)

6. Paul says that our life and freedom in Christ is meant to lead us to love others. How has your specific sexual sin struggle resulted in a lack of love toward others? What encouragement for change does this passage offer you?

7. Galatians 5:19 says that the "works of the flesh are evident," or obvious. In light of this, reflect again on last week's article, "God's Design for Sexuality." How are you increasingly seeing the obvious nature of your sexual sin and how it doesn't "fit" with God's design for sexual expression? In other words, how is God revealing it to be what it truly is—a turning away from him in order to pursue your own "broken cistern"?

8. Notice the wide variety of sins listed in verses 19–21, yet without any one sin being considered worse than the other. Notice also the fruit of the Holy Spirit in verses 22–23—the very character of Jesus being made manifest in our lives. Which of these fruit do you most desire to grow in, as a way of seeking to turn *to* God, and why?

Making It Personal (10 minutes)

God cares about what you do with your sexuality. Better yet, God is able to change you, as you grow in a lifestyle of turning from sinful patterns and turning toward him. God doesn't call sexual sin worse than other sins—but he *does* call it sin and an idolatrous turning away from him. Likewise, God doesn't label or identify us according to our sin, but sees us as in Christ (or not in Christ). The good news of the gospel of grace is that in Christ we become new creations, free of shame and forgiven of sin. Our lifelong journey includes learning how to turn from the works of the flesh as we learn to walk by the Spirit (Galatians 5:16).

Close your discussion time in prayer.

On Your Own (5 minutes)

1. Read Appendix B, "Broken Sexuality: What Happens When We Turn Away From God's Good Design" (p. 173), to gain more understanding into why sexual sin is a broken expression of God's good design.

2. Take the time to read and reflect upon Galatians 5:13–26 and Titus 2:11–14. What hope and encouragement do these passages offer you?

SESSION 6
THE FRUIT: UNDERSTANDING FEMALE HOMOSEXUALITY

KEY CONCEPT: When women turn to each other in relationally idolatrous ways, the sin of it is sometimes hard to recognize. After all, women are created to be nurturing, affectionate, and emotionally intimate . . . right? However, women are designed to be friends, sisters, and spiritual mentors or mothers to one another—not romantic pursuits, husband-replacements, or "mini-marriages" that mimic God's design for marriage. An idolatrous attraction and pull between women flows from the same place as that which fuels the woman who obsessively craves the emotional and/or sexual attention of men—her heart!

SESSION 6—THE FRUIT: UNDERSTANDING FEMALE HOMOSEXUALITY

Review and Reflect (15 minutes)

Open your session in prayer. Review last week's Key Concept, and then discuss the questions that follow:

Last Week's Key Concept: In contrast to God's design for sex, sexual sin is the fruit of a self-ruled and idolatrous heart. Sexual activity outside marriage (with women or men)—with self (masturbation), with someone else's spouse, sexual fantasy, and the viewing and reading of pornography—are ways women seek sexual pleasure and emotional comfort outside God's wise boundaries. These behaviors are the fruit of a heart living against God's created design for sexual expression.

1. How were you encouraged, or challenged, by Galatians 5:13–26 and Titus 2:11–14?

2. Reflect again on the article, "Broken Sexuality." What insights did you have as you read? What hope do you have in the realization that while the fall has impacted every part of us (including our sexuality), we have everything we need through Jesus to escape our sinful desires and live as godly women?

Exploring the Key Issue (60 minutes)

Read this week's Key Concept and the section that follows. Then, discuss the questions that come afterward.

Key Concept: When women turn to each other in relationally idolatrous ways, the sin of it is sometimes hard to recognize. After all, women are created to be nurturing, affectionate, and emotionally intimate . . . right? However, women are designed to be friends, sisters, and spiritual mentors or mothers to one another—not romantic pursuits, husband-replacements, or "mini-marriages" that mimic God's design for marriage. An idolatrous attraction and pull between women flows from the same place as that which fuels the woman who obsessively craves the emotional and/or sexual attention of men—her heart!

Session 5 explored some of the ways women dig their own "broken cisterns" (Jeremiah 2:13) in sexually sinful ways. Whenever we step outside God's design for any area of life, whether it's a sexual sin or any other, we express our sin nature. Homosexuality is yet one more way that women experience brokenness in their sexuality, acting upon their desires in sinful behavior and thoughts.

The spectrum of experience is wide when considering emotional and sexual attraction to other women. On one end are emotionally enmeshed and dependent relationships that have a romantic or sensual feel to them, which is a form of idolatry; on the other end, a woman embraces a gay identity and pursues a homosexual relationship (or several).

What does the Bible say about homosexuality? To understand the message of Scripture concerning homosexuality, or *any* area of temptation and sin, it's necessary to understand the whole counsel of God's Word. To develop a position by merely looking up singled-out verses from a Bible concordance is not only unwise, but poor teaching. The scope of this session prevents us from doing an exhaustive study of God's Word. The following is a concise summary of what the Bible teaches, with a few key passages for each point. (For further resources concerning homosexuality, visit the Harvest USA website at www. harvestusa.org.)

a. God is Creator of all, and has a design for all of life. This includes our sexuality (Genesis 1–2; Psalm 24:1–2; John 1:3; Colossians 1:16).

b. Sin has impacted all of creation, including people and our sexuality. Our bodies, desires, thoughts, minds, wills, capacity to do what is good and right, and the ability to discern good from evil have all been polluted by sin. What was meant to be natural to us—the image of God in us—has now become very *un*natural to us. We are born in sin, and therefore it is now our sinful nature that feels natural, easy, and comfortable to us. In fact, it seems to actually *be* us. Jesus came as Savior, Healer, and Redeemer, offering us new life through the forgiveness of sin, and the power to deny our sinful nature and live a life of Christlikeness (2 Peter 1:3–4; Romans 13:12–14; Galatians 5:16).

c. Homosexuality is sexual sin, as God has designed sexual activity to be contained in the marriage relationship, defined as one woman with one man for life. Nowhere in the Bible is homosexuality encouraged or blessed; rather, whenever sexual expression is encouraged in the Scriptures, it always refers to a marriage covenant between a man and a woman (Genesis 1–2; Ephesians 5:22–32; Matthew 19:4–6; Romans 1:24–27; 1 Corinthians 6:9).

d. Emotional lust and mental fantasy are forms of idolatry. Replacing love and worship for Jesus with a craving for deep and intense connection with another person (same or opposite gender, often called emotional dependency) is also sin. Emotional idolatry leads us to use people rather than truly love them. Mental fantasy is another way we replace the Creator with the creation, seeking life in a broken cistern (Jeremiah 2:11–13; Romans 12:9–10; 1 Peter 1:22)! Women with same-sex attraction tend to have a deep desire to find an emotional home through a deep and intense connection with another woman. This craving to be loved, accepted, valued, needed, and pursued is, at its heart, the same drive that fuels a heterosexually attracted woman to lust for the emotional and sexual attentions and affections of men!

e. Same-sex attraction (i.e., a *temptation* toward other women that may be emotional, romantic, and/or sexual in nature) is not sin unless acted upon in thought and/or behavior. First Corinthians 10:13–14 encourages us that *all* temptation is common to humankind! Temptation is a form of suffering, and a trial through which Christ offers a way of escape. Thus, we're given the opportunity to participate in Christ's sufferings as we bring our temptations, disordered desires, and broken hearts to him.

f. The concept of a "gay identity" is a newer development that gained popularity in the 20th century. Homosexual desire, temptation, and activity have been around as long as any heterosexual sins and temptations. However, there has been a shift to placing these desires and temptations into the category of *orientation* or *identity*—something that is said to be inborn and unchangeable, "who I am." Labeling or defining oneself on the basis of attractions, feelings, or behavior, is an attempt to define the essence of a person in a way that circumvents what Scripture says about that issue. In other words, by saying "I was born gay," one can then interpret everything Scripture says about homosexuality as no longer being applicable, because it is thought that the writers of Scripture were not "educated" enough to understand the issue in the way we do now. But to see life from a biblical perspective and live within God's design is to acknowledge that God's Word nowhere affirms or encourages such self-identification. The essence of who we are, our identity, is grounded in how God sees us. He identifies us as his people, or those who aren't his people—as sons and daughters in the family of God because we are "in Christ", or as people without Christ and outside his family (1 Peter 2:10; 1 John 5:12). Our identity, therefore, comes from our relationship with God.

3. Do you disagree with any of the above? As you read, did you have any insights that you hadn't considered before? Explain.

4. Read the following questions and text and discuss together as a group.

What has been your understanding of homosexuality or why someone might be gay? Do you think it's possible for someone to change—to be free of homosexuality or same-sex attractions? Why or why not? These are loaded questions within both the psychological and Christian communities. There is significant debate over whether change is possible. But as with any disordered desire or pattern of sin, change is absolutely possible through Jesus Christ (2 Peter 1:3–4)! However, the Bible does not give us the guarantee that we'll be completely free of temptation while we live on this earth. Temptation, and the battle against ungodly desires and thoughts, will be a lifelong battle for all of us! However, over time, as we become conformed to Christ and grow in maturity as his followers, the intensity, frequency, and draw toward sin diminishes. This is a process unique to each follower. Some same-sex-tempted women experience a complete shift in their desires from women to men, or to *one man* who will become their husband; others don't. But testimonies abound of women who are living godly, sexually pure lives, even as the attraction to women is still present. The ultimate goal is never a generalized heterosexuality but **holiness** (growing in learning how to live my life according to God's design)—as it is for all followers of Christ! Some women may not ever experience what is commonly called "heterosexual attraction" but *may* develop an attraction to *one* man whom God is calling them to marry. This "specific person" attraction might be called being *husband-sexual*: experiencing an emotional, spiritual, and sexual attraction to the one God calls a woman to enter into a marriage covenant with! This is, in fact, what God's design for marriage is: that two would forsake all others to enter into a lifelong marriage of faithfulness and devotion to Christ and one another.

5. If you're a woman who struggles with same-sex temptations, how have you experienced feeling shame, isolation, or fear when it comes to sharing your struggle with others? What have been the messages you've heard from Christians regarding homosexuality?

6. Emotional dependency or relational idolatry could be defined this way: *believing that the presence of a person and the ongoing emotional connection and attachment I have with that person is necessary for security and well-being.*[1] What role has emotional dependency played in your own life and relationships? How does it lead us to using people rather than loving them? (Read these passages for insight: Mark 10:45; Romans 12:9–12; 2 Corinthians 5:14–15.)

Making It Personal (10 minutes)

Sessions 5 and 6 are just an overview of the different ways that women are tempted and struggle with sexual and relational sin. You might have been surprised at the similarity of all sexual sin, whether heterosexual or homosexual. At the core, sexual sin is a way women seek to find life in other people and sexual experiences. Women who are same-sex tempted may strive to find an emotional home in the arms and connection with another woman—but women who crave the sexual attentions of men are really doing the same thing. Likewise, those who are tempted and succumb to the more "solo sins" of pornography and masturbation seek refuge via the comfort and escape of the sexual experience.

No matter what the struggle, life as a follower of Jesus calls for obedience to his Word and to remain true to him and his ways. This happens as we grow in understanding ourselves, our temptations, our sexuality, and our desires through a biblical lens. God's Word brings clarity and helps us to have a transformation in our thinking, which leads us to a deeper understanding of our identity in Christ.

On Your Own (5 minutes)

The next session will begin to unpack other elements of the Harvest USA Tree Model, beginning with the soil. So take time this week to reflect on your fruit, and to prepare for the sessions to come. Review Sessions 2–5, especially Session 3.

SESSION 7
UNDERSTANDING OUR SOIL

KEY CONCEPT: Influences outside of our control, while not determinative, can have a strong shaping force upon us. These influences are the "soil" of the Tree Model. None of us chooses the family or culture we're born into, our gender, our body type, personality, or the specific forms of blessing, suffering, and sin that may come at us as we live in this fallen world. Generally, our family dynamics are a combination of positive and negative experiences that may include both rich blessing and profound suffering. Understanding how our views of gender, sex, relationships, blessing, suffering, pain, personal identity, and God (among others) were shaped by our unique soil can help us understand why we tend toward certain patterns of relating, emotional response, and coping.

SESSION 7—UNDERSTANDING OUR SOIL

Review and Reflect (15 minutes)

Open your session in prayer. Review last week's Key Concept, and then discuss the questions that follow:

Last Week's Key Concept: When women turn to each other in relationally idolatrous ways, the sin of it is sometimes hard to recognize. After all, women are created to be nurturing, affectionate, and emotionally intimate . . . right? However, women are designed to be friends, sisters, and spiritual mentors or mothers to one another—not romantic pursuits, husband-replacements, or partners in "mini-marriages" that mimic God's design for marriage. An idolatrous attraction and pull between women flows from the same place as that which fuels the woman who obsessively craves the emotional and/or sexual attention of men—her heart!

1. What new questions, if any, came up about Session 6 and homosexuality?

2. How are you discovering that no matter what the sin struggle, we're much more alike than we are different? What have you learned about God's design for sexuality, the broken ways we experience it, and the hope we have for change through Jesus?

Exploring the Key Issue (60 minutes)

Read this week's Key Concept and the paragraph that follows, aloud. Then, discuss the questions afterward.

Key Concept: Influences outside our control, while not determinative, can have a strong shaping force upon us. These influences are the "soil" of the Tree Model. None of us chooses the family or culture we're born into, our gender, our body type, personality, or the specific forms of blessing, suffering, and sin that may come at us as we live in this fallen world. Generally, our family dynamics are a combination of positive and negative experiences that may include both rich blessing and profound suffering. Understanding how our views of gender, sex, relationships, blessing, suffering, pain, personal identity, and God (among others) were shaped by our unique soil can help us understand why we tend toward certain patterns of relating, emotional response, and coping.

Session 2 introduced the concept of our soil influences. In this session, we begin a more in-depth study of the Tree Model with an overview of our soil influences. As we begin, it's important to remember that these influences are not *determinative*; they don't *cause* us to act in a certain way. However they can, and often do, exert strong shaping power upon us. They shape the way we interpret life and impact the development of our worldviews (or beliefs) regarding all of life, including God, people, relationships, our gender, the opposite gender, sexuality, and the way this world works.

Read the following and discuss the questions.

3. The Tree Model helps us to understand how our life patterns (habits of thought, behavior, emotions, desires, beliefs, and attitudes) developed. Soil influences encompass not only how we've experienced life in the past, but presently; not only events but "givens," such as being female, our body type, our particular talents, gifts, and personality. Our lives today have been impacted by the way we've experienced and responded to life previously; our godly and ungodly life patterns have developed in part due to our godly and ungodly responses to life as it's come at us, often out of our control. Do you agree with these thoughts? Explain your answer.

4. Sometimes women accept labels or identities for themselves based on sin done against us. What examples can you think of? (For example, a woman who has suffered sexual abuse may identify herself as "damaged goods.")

5. What's life been like for you as a woman? Have you enjoyed being female? Have you ever wished you were born male? Explain your answers.

6. A popular saying is "The devil made me do it!" and is a tongue-in-cheek way to blame sinful behavior solely upon Satan. The Bible actually does address the reality of how the devil is a very real enemy! Read Ephesians 6:10–12 together and share what it teaches us in regards to our struggles, as well as how the kingdom of darkness is a soil influence. In your experience as a Christian, have you tended to overemphasize or underemphasize the reality of spiritual warfare as a normal part of being a follower of Christ?

7. A significant soil we are "planted" in is our family. Our home environment was the first place we learned what relationships, marriage, gender, family, and so many other things looked like. What are 4–5 words or phrases that describe

how your experience of family was positive and/or negative? (Session 8 will explore family dynamics in more detail.)

Making It Personal (10 minutes)

Read the following section aloud:

As we delve into our soil, we begin to realize that our sexual and relational behaviors didn't just fall out of the sky! There are identifiable patterns we can unearth, and we must start by understanding how our hearts (seed) were impacted by our soil. We will grow in being able to see our sexual issues for what they are as we understand our soil-influenced hearts. The next several sessions will examine specific impactful events, people, and/or circumstances that have had a shaping influence.

As you progress through the soil sessions, some questions might seem redundant. However, it's important to tell and retell your story. Each retelling of your story is an opportunity to unearth a different viewpoint or emotion. As you do so, you'll come to deal with these new emotions or perspectives on a deeper level of healing than before. Further, don't underestimate the power of telling and retelling your stories in the presence of others. You never know how the Lord might open the eyes of someone else's heart in your group via *your* story!

On Your Own (5 minutes)

It's challenging to look honestly at our lives and the painful experiences we've had. Many people live their entire lives in denial and avoidance of these things. However, while God's wisdom will never lead us to morbid introspection, God invites us to ask him to search us out (Psalm 139:23–24), so that we may be led away from our own destructive paths and onto his everlasting paths of faith, obedience, and wholeness.

Many believers have found the book of Psalms to be one of the most comforting books in the Bible because of its unashamed honesty in describing the sorrows and heartaches of human experience. People often don't realize that the Bible really *does* speak into the very painful, gritty experiences of life on this earth!

1. Read the following passages in Psalms, and reflect on how your life experiences mirror what the psalmist says:

Heartache: Psalms 25:16–18; 31:9–10; 34:18; 147:3

Betrayal and abandonment: Psalms 31:11–12; 38:9–11; 142

Traumatic and life-threatening circumstances: Psalms 23:4; 35:1–3; 63

Hateful enemies: Psalms 3:1–2, 6; 25:19; 41:5; 59

Broken families: Psalms 38:11; 69:8

2. Reflect and respond to the following questions regarding family dynamics:

a. What was your home life like as you grew up? Who raised you? What was your experience of family?

b. What do you appreciate about your home life and experience of family, or primary caregivers as you grew up? What are aspects of your upbringing and family life that are painful and confusing?

c. What are you thankful for as you consider your mom and dad? What was your relationship like with them, if you knew them? What is painful for you as you think of your experience of being a daughter? And of being a sister if you had siblings?

d. As your parents/caregivers raised you, they like you, were needy sinners desperately dependent upon Jesus Christ for grace, mercy, forgiveness, and wisdom. In what ways have you been aware of this as an adult, and how has this shaped the way you view your parents/caregivers?

e. Remembering and considering the impact of our past experiences, including our family of origin, is something that God's people did as well. Read Psalm 106 then reflect on the following and journal about any new insights.

Psalm 106:6–12 recounts how the Israelites said, "Both we and our fathers have sinned; we have committed iniquity; we have done wickedness. Our fathers, when they were in Egypt, did not consider your wondrous works; they did not remember the abundance of your steadfast love, but rebelled by the sea, at the Red Sea. Yet . . . he saved them from the hand of the foe and redeemed them from the power of the enemy. And the waters covered their adversaries; not one of them was left. Then they believed his words; they sang his praise."

Psalm 106 goes on to tell of the past sin of family members and how God responded and related to them. The key is that, as the Israelites considered their history, it was done from a God-centric lens: *What was God doing? How did he respond? How did the sins of their fathers show rebellion, ultimately against their loving God? And how have they (who are remembering the Lord's past faithfulness and their family's past unfaithfulness) continued in their own sin against God?*

This is one of many portions of Scripture that guide us in how to view our pasts. The Israelites expressed a clear understanding that their forefathers *and they* had experienced the blessing and gracious love of God, and that their forefathers *and they* had committed sin against God. We don't think about painful family dynamics, sin done against us by our parents and other significant people, heartbreaking losses, and other hard "soils" for the sake of knowing them alone, or to blame our sinful choices on what happened to us! We are to follow the model of the Israelites: acknowledging our history's impact upon us, and how our response to it was either pleasing or displeasing to God; how our interpretation of past events was grounded in a Jesus-centric lens, or a me-centric lens; how we have chosen and "watered" holy or sinful patterns of life. Gaining awareness into how *we've allowed* our history to impact us assists us in understanding how our present sin struggles and patterns of life developed. Our relational and sexual sin patterns didn't just happen to us. We have chosen and watered them over time as our hearts responded to and made interpretations about life in a fallen and broken world. Our pasts do not define us, nor have they caused us to willfully choose any of the relational or sexual sins we struggle with now. The hopeful news of Jesus Christ, is that his truth about life, including our personal experiences, is *the truth* that sets us free (see John 8:31–32)!

(***Note:*** *Sessions 8 and 9 are structured for a 2-hour meeting. Talk to your group leader if this presents a challenge for you!*)

SESSION 8
THE SOIL: FAMILY DYNAMICS—ROLES, RULES, AND RELATIONAL PATTERNS

KEY CONCEPT: God designed families, and our home environment, to have a profound impact in our lives—and they always do! Within our families (or home environment) we learn (through spoken and unspoken messages) about relationships, spirituality, marriage, emotions, communication, sexuality, security, and so much more. Families generally function and relate to one another based on a variety of dynamics, three of which are the roles, rules, and relational patterns that are embedded in the fabric of a family's life. As we grow in awareness of how these soil dynamics existed in our home environment, *and the meaning we assigned to them*, we gain insight into why and how we developed certain beliefs (shoots) about how life is supposed to work.

SESSION 8—THE SOIL: FAMILY DYNAMICS— ROLES, RULES, AND RELATIONAL PATTERNS

Review and Reflect (15 minutes)

Open your session in prayer. Review last week's Key Concept, and then discuss the questions that follow:

Last Week's Key Concept: Influences outside our control, while not determinative, can have a strong shaping force upon us. These influences are the "soil" of the Tree Model. None of us chooses the family or culture we're born into, our gender, our body type, personality, or the specific forms of blessing, suffering, and sin that may come at us as we live in this fallen world. Generally, our family dynamics are a combination of positive and negative experiences that may include both rich blessing and profound suffering. Understanding how our views of gender, sex, relationships, blessing, suffering, pain, personal identity, and God (among others) were shaped by our unique soil can help us understand why we tend toward certain patterns of relating, emotional response, and coping.

1. What encouraged, comforted, or challenged you as you read the passages from the Psalms this past week? How did you connect your experiences of pain and suffering with the words of the psalmist?

2. What insights did you gain from the reflective questions about your family?

3. What fears or concerns do you feel as we prepare to explore family dynamics more deeply?

Exploring the Key Issue (75 minutes)

Read this week's Key Concept:

Key Concept: God designed families, and our home environment, to have a profound impact in our lives—and they always do! Within our families (or home environment) we learn (through spoken and unspoken messages) about relationships, spirituality, marriage, emotions, communication, sexuality, security, and so much more. Families generally function and relate to one another based on a variety of dynamics, three of which are the roles, rules, and relational patterns that are embedded in the fabric of a family's life. As we grow in awareness of how these soil dynamics existed in our home environment, *and the meaning we assigned to them*, we gain insight into why and how we developed certain beliefs (shoots) about how life is supposed to work.

Discuss the following.

4. Divide up the following passages among group members. Take a few minutes to read your given passage silently, and then share what it teaches about God's design for family life.

a. Proverbs 22:6
b. Ephesians 5:22–30
c. Ephesians 6:1–4
d. Colossians 3:18–21

Read the following silently then discuss the question.

Roles and Rules

In God's design, families are meant to be a theater for his glory and a classroom for instruction and nurture on how to do life. God's intention is that families be a signpost that displays who God is and what it looks like to love others. His design is that within our families we would "work out our salvation," learning how to apply godliness to all the ways we experience life on earth. As already discussed, this world is impacted by sin, and thus there is no family in human history void of dysfunction. No family has ever had perfect, sin-free dynamics regarding communication, conflict resolution, affection, emotional honesty, wise nurture, and boundaries. Because this is true, it's important to understand how our family experiences have influenced and perhaps distorted our views in these areas and many more.

Most families, if not all, have spoken and unspoken rules for how the family functions, and the roles family members fill to keep the family dynamic in place. Consider the following:

Rules: Family rules dictate how members of the family interact and behave, both verbally and nonverbally. These are often unspoken and subtle, but not always. For example:

Don't talk or . . . talk about everything.

Don't trust.

Don't feel or . . . let everyone know how you feel all the time.

It's not OK to be needy and weak.

It's not OK to cry or hurt.

Deny or minimize conflict.

Never criticize or disagree.

Keep peace at any cost.

Don't air the dirty laundry.

Never discuss family secrets.

The family must stand together, family is always first.

5. What rules are you aware of, that undergirded the way your family functioned? How have you continued to live under these rules as an adult in your relationships with women? Men? What helpful rules did your family have?

Read the following and discuss the questions that follow.

Roles: These are ways a person learns to act within the family—the specific part she plays in the drama and functioning of the family system. Roles often come as a child adapts to a number of factors. They're a way of fitting in or coping with the family or with a particular family member; they also serve to keep the others' roles in place. For example:

The Doer—is a performance-driven person who consistently must do what is "right."

The Wall Flower/Chameleon—is the child or parent who "goes with the flow," because it is safer to not draw attention to oneself. She tends to avoid conflict and get lost within the family.

The Martyr—is a doer, but must let everyone know *what* she's doing (serving, giving, etc.) and what personal sacrifice is being made as she's doing it.

The Peacemaker —keeps peace between family members, and often feels responsible for everyone. In Christian families, a *Peacemaker* may also grow into the role of *Spiritual Advisor* or *Family Pastor,* taking on responsibility for the spiritual well-being of the family.

The Scapegoat—is blamed for everything, and is often viewed as the "black sheep" or troublemaker in the family.

The Clown—uses humor in reaction to uncomfortable moments, and often is expected to break the tension with a joke.

The Caregiver—assumes the caretaker role, parental role, and perhaps a spousal role.

The Princess/Daddy's Girl—can do no wrong and is seen as the darling of the family.

The Surrogate Spouse—takes on the emotional role of husband or wife to her father and/or mother, being confided in and depended upon inappropriately, and sometimes sexually misused/abused.

6. What role did you fill in your family? Maybe it's a combination of some items in this list, or there's a better descriptive word for it. How do you see yourself still living in light of that role as an adult? What roles did other family members live out—and perhaps continue to live out? Do you think your relational patterns now were influenced by the role(s) you lived out in your family? If yes, how so?

7. What roles are there for followers of Jesus to live out? Putting it another way, even if we learned and continue to live out certain roles in our relationships, what do you think Jesus would say are the most important roles for his followers to live out?

Read the following and discuss the questions.

Relational Patterns

We've discussed the idea of how we each have a "pattern of life" that has developed over time. This pattern includes how we respond to conflict, how we express our feelings, how we both pursue and avoid people, and the roles we live out in our relationships. A third family dynamic that shapes us is the way we learned to relate to other people. Let's consider a passage of Scripture that teaches us what is to be avoided and pursued in godly relationships. We'll use it to discern what relational patterns we have learned (perhaps unconsciously!) that honor God; we'll also see how ungodly ways of relating may have been modeled for us. Remember, our goal isn't to assign blame or to become discouraged! Rather, we want to learn to love and relate as Jesus loved and related, and now he enables us to imitate him through the Holy Spirit.

8. Read Colossians 3:1–17 aloud as a group, then write your responses to the questions which follow. When done writing your answers, discuss your insights together as a group.

a. What types of behavior and relating are mentioned in verses 5–9 which Paul says we are to "put to death"? Were any of these active in your home as you grew up? Would you say any are presently active in your life?

b. What types of behavior and relational patterns are mentioned in verses 12–17? Notice that Paul says we are to "put [these] on" because we are "God's chosen ones, holy and beloved." Were any of these modeled for you in your home growing up? How have you walked in them yourself? Did you experience the opposite of these relational qualities in your home life? If yes, how so?

c. Now consider the relational and sexual sin patterns with which you are struggling presently. Being out of control sexually or addicted to pornography and/or masturbation did not happen overnight. Generally women who are same-sex tempted (through habitually being emotionally dependent with a woman or involved sexually with women) took lots of mini-steps in this direction before recognizing they had a problem. Look back at your answers for (a) and (b) and consider the history of your sexual or relational struggle. Over the course of time, what types of behaviors have you "put off" that

Christ wanted you to *put on*? What types of behaviors were you putting on (participating in), that Christ wanted you to "put to death"?

Making It Personal (25 minutes)

Reading the following section aloud:

Sexual sin, and the broken cisterns associated with it, is the manifestation of sinful, weak human hearts that have not learned to navigate life in godly, healthy ways. The emotional comfort and sexual pleasure gained through encounters with women, men, self, or pornography are sinful coping strategies for dealing with life. Of course, there are many ways people self-medicate, but sexual and relational sins provide an easy escape path for women who have never learned healthy relating.

As we journey to honestly face how sin has developed in our lives, consider this wonderful prayer—one we've looked at before—from Psalm 139:23–24: "Search me, O God, and know my heart! Try me and know my thoughts! And see if there be any grievous way in me, and lead me in the way everlasting!" We can honestly reflect upon our own sinful strategies for dealing with life and, in doing so, examine the impact of our families upon our lives. He alone can lead us in a new way of viewing ourselves as women, as sexual beings, and as females in relationships of integrity with both genders.

We need to remember, too, that our reactions to good things can easily nurture lust and selfishness in our hearts! When we experience goodness and receive good things, we can develop a demanding spirit that leads to sinful attitudes. Those attitudes bear fruit in sinful patterns of living, including our relationships and expression of sexuality. For example, if we received significant flattery or praise for legitimate (or illegitimate) behaviors, we may later live for flattery or praise from others. Or if we grew up always getting what we wanted, we may have a demanding spirit that must feel comfort all the time. Any time

God reveals sin to us, it is an invitation to come to his throne of grace, which he says we can approach with confidence to receive mercy and help in our time of need (Hebrews 4:16)!

Close the time in prayer.

On Your Own (5 minutes)

1. Moms and dads are a significant soil influence in our development. Take some time to journal out any insights you've gained about how your mother (or if you were not raised by your mom, a significant maternal-like caregiver you may have had) helped or hindered you in learning how to express feelings, what she taught you about being a woman, and what you learned from her regarding men and how to relate to them. Do the same for your father or a significant paternal-like caregiver if you were not raised by your father. If you were not raised by either of your parents, what influence has this had on you that you're aware of? Regardless of how you experienced being parented, consider reading David Powlison's excellent article, "What if Your Father Didn't Love You?"[2]

2. Within the sphere of family dynamics, we can also gain insight into our own patterns through considering the boundaries and messages that were a part of our home environment. Read the mini-article below and the reflective questions that follow. Journal about any insights you gain from your reading and reflection. These will not be discussed in the next session; however they will be helpful for you to gain more insight into the development of your "manner of life." (See Session 7 for review!) Generally, adults tend to repeat the patterns (godly and ungodly) they learned as children. Without the gracious intervention of the Lord and his truth and love, we would all continue in worldly patterns of expressing ourselves sexually and relationally. Ask the Lord to "search you out" and lead you in his ways as you consider these questions.

The Soil: Family Dynamics - Boundaries and Messages

There are many family dynamics that constitute the "soil influence" of family. Along with rules, roles, and relational patterns there are boundaries and messages. These refer to boundaries that were or weren't in existence, and the spoken and unspoken messages about matters such as gender, sibling favoritism, and what were praiseworthy or unpraiseworthy characteristics.

Read the descriptions that follow and the questions. Journal out what you think the most impacting boundaries and messages were in your family.

Boundaries: Healthy boundaries provide a sense of security, comfort, safety, trust, intimacy, affection . . . the list is endless. Lack of boundaries, or overly tight boundaries, can lead those in a family to grow up without the safety of healthy, expressed love and nurture that a family is meant to provide. Because they are a group of sinners, families fall within the spectrum between rigid boundaries and no boundaries at all.

Messages: These are the things most frequently communicated regarding gender categories and their roles. They're the stereotypes our particular family latched onto—"the way it is." Examples:

- A woman always needs a man, regardless of his behavior or attitude, even if it's abusive or controlling.
- Boys will be boys.
- A boy can engage in sex and/or masturbation, because that's how they're made.
- A girl must never have sex but must remain a virgin for her husband.
- A girl is either a virgin or a whore/slut.
- Males are to be the leaders, because they're superior.
- Whatever a man thinks, decides, or feels is right.
- Women are weak and emotional, rather than strong and logical like men.
- Women are inferior/superior to men.
- To be different from your family (in personality or thinking) is wrong and a sign of disobedience and/or disrespect.

a. Describe the messages or stereotypes taught within your family about men and their roles, and about women and their roles.

b. What boundaries, or lack of them, did your family have concerning things like personal space, involvement in each other's lives, and sharing confidences? How has this shaped the way you view boundaries now?

c. Read Romans 8:12–17. This is one of many passages that helps us understand the idea of being a child—or in our case, a *daughter*—of God. As we consider the dynamics in our earthly family, it's important to remember that in Christ, we are born into God's family, a family of brothers and sisters with one father, God. Reflect on this and other passages that teach about the family of God (such as Romans 12:9–21; Ephesians 5:1–2; 1 John 3:1–3, 16–18; and 1 John 4:7). Ask God to give you insight into what it means to be *God's daughter* and a sister to other believers.

3. Read 1 Peter 1:6–7. Peter says that through the trials we face in this life (which includes painful family experiences), our faith is proven and honor comes to Jesus Christ. How do you think honor can come to Jesus as you face the trials that have come via your family background, and take steps of faith to live with your heart set on him and the hope he offers for healing and change? How is God making you aware of your own need for healing, as well as your need to extend forgiveness? (The Bible speaks often of suffering and that it is normal for us while we live in this fallen world. Consider reading these passages to gain a fuller understanding of how a biblical lens views trials: John 15:18–16:1, 33; Acts 7:54–8:3; 2 Corinthians 1:1–11; Hebrews 11:32–40; James 1:1–4.)

SESSION 9
THE SOIL: TRAUMATIC PAIN

KEY CONCEPT: When we experience traumatic and painful events such as abuse, loss, and abandonment, we respond and react to a world that is unsafe and unpredictable. As we understand how these profoundly painful experiences have impacted us, and the ways we responded to them, we gain additional insight into how our idolatrous ways of relating to people and life developed. This wisdom guides us in turning from false comforts to the True Comforter, Jesus Christ.

SESSION 9—THE SOIL: TRAUMATIC PAIN

Review and Reflect (15 minutes)

Open your session in prayer. Review last week's Key Concept, and then discuss the questions that follow:

Last Week's Key Concept: God designed families, and our home environment, to have a profound impact in our lives—and they always do! Within our families (or home environment) we learn (through spoken and unspoken messages) about relationships, spirituality, marriage, emotions, communication, sexuality, security, and so much more. Families generally function and relate to one another based on a variety of dynamics, three of which are the roles, rules, and relational patterns that are embedded in the fabric of a family's life. As we grow in awareness of how these soil dynamics existed in our home environments, *and the meaning we assigned to them*, we gain insight into why and how we developed certain beliefs (shoots) about how life is supposed to work.

1. What did you learn from your reading and reflection of the Bible passages in last week's homework (or others you found)? How do these truths encourage you about your spiritual identity?

2. What did God show you as you reflected upon 1 Peter 1:6–7, and other Bible passages that teach us about suffering and trials? What are you learning about the hope we have in/through Jesus in regards to experiences of suffering?

Exploring the Key Issue (75 minutes)

Read this week's Key Concept, and the passage that follows. Then, discuss the questions afterward.

Key Concept: When we experience traumatic and painful events such as abuse, loss, and abandonment, we respond and react to a world that is unsafe and unpredictable. As we understand how these profoundly painful experiences have impacted us, and the ways we responded to them, we gain additional insight into how our idolatrous ways of relating to people and life developed. This wisdom guides us in turning from false comforts to the True Comforter, Jesus Christ.

Psalm 57 was written by David in reference to the abuse and murderous hatred he suffered through Saul, a man who had been a role model and leader for him. First Samuel 22 and 24 chronicle two occasions of David fleeing Saul's hatred toward him. It was during one of these instances that David wrote Psalm 57, a powerful example of a godly person crying out in pain to God for help.

> Have mercy on me, O God, have mercy on me,
>   for in you my soul takes refuge.
> I will take refuge in the shadow of your wings
>   until the disaster has passed.
> I cry out to God Most High,
>   to God, who fulfills his purpose for me.
> He sends from heaven and saves me,
>   rebuking those who hotly pursue me;
>   God sends his love and his faithfulness.
> I am in the midst of lions;
>   I lie among ravenous beasts—
> men whose teeth are spears and arrows,
>   whose tongues are sharp swords.
> Be exalted, O God, above the heavens;
>   let your glory be over all the earth.
> They spread a net for my feet—
>   I was bowed down in distress.

They dug a pit in my path—
 but they have fallen into it themselves.
My heart is steadfast, O God,
 my heart is steadfast;
 I will sing and make music.
Awake, my soul!
 Awake, harp and lyre!
 I will awaken the dawn.
I will praise you, O Lord, among the nations;
 I will sing of you among the peoples.
For great is your love, reaching to the heavens;
 your faithfulness reaches to the skies.
Be exalted, O God, above the heavens;
 let your glory be over all the earth. (Psalm 57:1–11 NIV)

Traumatic experiences come in a variety of forms, and abuse can be emotional, physical, sexual, and/or spiritual. As we assess these events and the feelings that often surface during such assessment, it's important to be emotionally honest. This honesty means that we face and feel the emotions rather than denying or minimizing them, and at the same time gain awareness of how we've sought to destructively soothe the pain associated with those memories. This is a healing process that takes time. But according to God's Word, the healing is real!

Types of trauma and abuse

Death—of parent(s), children, siblings, closes relatives, friends, mentors, spiritual leaders.

Loss—of relationship through divorce, abandonment, betrayal, rejection; *loss* of health through illness or injury; *loss* of independence through physical disability, financial struggles or through needing to be a caregiver.

Physical Abuse—includes inappropriate punishment, hitting, slapping, pushing, grabbing, punishing out of anger, physical neglect, and/or abandonment.

Sexual abuse—includes exposure to sexual things, being treated as a surrogate spouse, vaginal penetration, touching, exposure to nudity, rape, flirting, over-interest in sexuality and/or body parts, staring, incest, oral sex, anal sex. "Sexual abuse is any contact or interaction (visual, verbal, or psychological) between a child/adolescent and an adult when the child/adolescent is being used for the sexual stimulation of the perpetrator or any other person."[3] Sexual abuse can also happen between adults.

Emotional Abuse—includes verbal abuse, criticism of gender, body or style, profanity, manipulation, screaming, shunning, shaming, harassment, name calling, no expression of affection, lack of intimacy and nurturing, lack of listening and touch, lack of interest, enmeshed relationships.

Spiritual Abuse—includes teachings that are manipulative; teachings that emphasize an angry God who's "out to get you"; using Scripture or religious teaching to gain power/control over others, to make others feel like a failure, unworthy, without choice, and/or powerless.

3. As you reflect on your life, what have been some of the most painful, and life-impacting losses you have faced? Did you experience comfort from anyone as you faced these losses? If yes, how so? If no, how did you seek to comfort yourself?

4. Are you an abuse survivor? If so, what are you willing to share with the group about your experience? Avoid graphic detail, but be honest about your feelings.

5. What's your response to this quote: "But abuse victims are notorious for ignoring or mislabeling how we are really feeling. Reflecting on our feelings, in addition to just our thoughts, can be a helpful way of breaking through our denial"[4]?

6. Are you aware of any ways these abusive events shaped your view(s) of the following: God, relationships/sex, men, women, yourself, the world?

7. Do you think you can trust God to lead you through facing your abuse and into healing and change? Why or why not? What would you like to say to God regarding your abuse?

Read the following and discuss the questions that follow.

"The Cycle of Abuse," developed by Sarah Lipp, describes a typical path of response by those who have suffered sexual abuse. When a child is abused, it is an act of betrayal. The perpetrator is often someone known to the victim, and thus her world is no longer safe. The people she expects to protect her are either involved in the abuse or do nothing about it (either because of denial or ignorance). The result inside the girl's heart is often a tragic cycle of response.

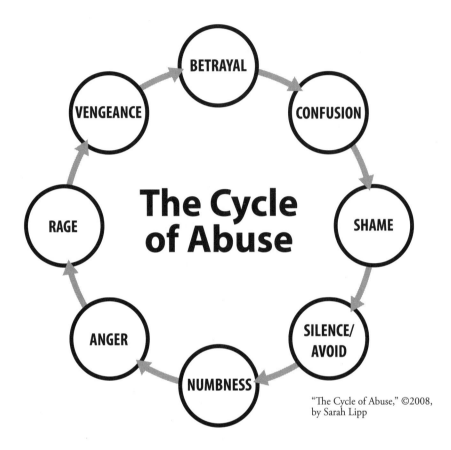

The Cycle of Abuse

BETRAYAL

CONFUSION

VENGEANCE

SHAME

RAGE

SILENCE/ AVOID

ANGER

NUMBERS

"The Cycle of Abuse," ©2008, by Sarah Lipp

Review the cycle and the descriptions of each phase below. Share how you see your own patterns of response and relating represented. Your homework for the next session will be to reflect more personally on these cycle components.

Betrayal—The first part of the cycle is when the abuse takes place. Feelings of betrayal and a profound sense of hurt settle in. Often, the victim becomes stuck in the same modes of interpretation and response that were present at the time of abuse.

Confusion—The victim thinks, "I thought he/she loved me," or, "I thought I was special but yet I feel violated and used." Perhaps there is confusion over what just happened. She knows it was wrong but can't verbalize or articulate what exactly occurred.

Shame—The victim feels dirty, guilty, and embarrassed: "Something is wrong with *me*."

Silence/Avoid—The victim says to herself, "No one will believe me. People will reject me if they knew what I did. It must be my fault. It will go away. I am powerless to change it." Many times the victim will deny the severity of what occurred or is still occurring.

Numbness—The victim disengages from her longing for anyone to ever really know her, now that she has this "dirty little secret." She shuts down her desires for love, acceptance, and to be special to someone. Ambivalence is prevalent; there is a conflict of ideas and attitudes. This inner conflict stems from the horror of the abuse experienced alongside perhaps "comforting" emotions or physical pleasure. "I felt pleasure, yet I feel dirty"; "I was terrified and it hurt so badly, but he told me he loved me and *that* felt good; "I felt pleasure yet felt powerless and betrayed at the same time. I desire his/her attention and I hate him/her." Ambivalence may lead to a sense of feeling responsible for what happened rather than seeing herself as a victim. This becomes her mode of survival.

Anger—The victim comes to a point of asking, "Why me?" or "Where was God or someone to protect me?" The victim feels robbed and very alone.

Rage—The victim develops an inner rage; a feeling that restores a sense of power and control. This is mostly internal; no one ever sees this deeply hidden feeling. Bitterness often settles in; yet, on the exterior, no one would truly realize the rage that is being felt.

Vengeance—The victim vows, "I will never let this happen again. I can never trust anyone"; "I will never put myself in a position to feel hurt, rejection, or abandonment"; or, "No one will protect or care for me, so I must do it myself."

While this sounds more like a progression, it in fact becomes a destructive cycle, because disappointment of some kind, (through unmet expectations, betrayal, rejection), is inevitable in all relationships. A woman may feel betrayed in present relationships, because all people are finite and fallen. No one treats her perfectly. An abuse victim, therefore, can continue to live in reaction to her past abuse, viewing all relationships with suspicion, criticalness, and an antagonistic attitude when someone gets too close. She thinks, "If I'm hurt in any way, I will hurt him back," or "I'll make her pay for hurting me."

Unfortunately, this often becomes a self-fulfilling prophecy. Whenever we experience hurt, we may lean toward seeking to betray (and sin against) the person that hurt us by cutting him or her off. This oftentimes results in the person eventually withdrawing and walking away from the relationship. Thus, we become people who refuse to extend forgiveness or to pursue full reconciliation with others and become isolated and self-sufficient. This relational pattern seems to make sense in light of an inner desire we may have to self-protect. However it actually is *self-serving* at the core and *doesn't* protect us, but rather insulates us from the love and blessing God may have for us via healthy relationships. Jesus Christ offers us a new way through the path of trusting him, not leaning on our own strategies for facing pain (Proverbs 3:5–6), and learning to move toward others in love (Colossians 3:12–13). Learning how to love and relate as the Lord desires is a process that we walk out, step by step and one circumstance at a time!

Making It Personal (25 minutes)

Read the following section silently. As you do, write your reflections in the space provided below.

"The LORD is near to the brokenhearted and saves the crushed in spirit" (Psalm 34:18). God is Father and Healer to the brokenhearted and bruised. No matter what the painful losses or abuse you may have suffered, he has hope for you. It's important that we don't allow this session to lead us to slide into self-pity or shame or to be tempted to despair. Facing our past abuse is an opportunity for personal growth and to know and experience the heart-healing that can only be found in Jesus. Facing sexual abuse challenges our beliefs about God and his provision and protection of us. Therefore, putting our past into perspective takes both emotional and spiritual work.

With the enabling grace of God, we can grow in faith and no longer be controlled by our past. We can attach the same significance to events that God does. There are many examples in Scripture of those who suffered circumstances out of their control, yet received the Lord's grace to turn around and put their past in a perspective that redeemed their suffering. Remember that Mary was confronted with becoming pregnant before marriage—before she even had sex, for that matter—knowing she would suffer societal abuse, become an outcast, and perhaps even be rejected by her husband-to-be. Nonetheless, she says, "Behold, I am the servant of the Lord; let it be to me according to your word" (Luke 1:38).

Think about Job, a man who lost everything—his children, land, money, reputation, friends, home, and physical well-being. Yet his summation of it all was, "The LORD gave, and the LORD has taken away; blessed be the name of the LORD" (Job 1:21).

Finally, don't forget Joseph, who was abused, rejected, and abandoned by his brothers; left for dead in a pit; sold into slavery; falsely accused and imprisoned; and forgotten by someone whose life he helped save. Joseph was able to view his painful experiences from God's perspective. Instead of rejecting his brothers or seeking revenge, Joseph chose forgiveness and mercy, reassuring them, "As for you, you meant evil against me, but God meant it for good, to bring it about that many people should be kept alive, as they are today" (Genesis 50:20).

These stories are not in God's Word to shame you, nor to discount your pain, but to give you hope! The trauma and suffering we encounter while we live in this world is *not* easily overcome. But when facing it by faith, it becomes a gospel opportunity. You can move through the healing process by holding onto the hope of Philippians 1:6, "that he who began a good work in you will bring it to completion at the day of Jesus Christ." God sees and knows you, and he is rescuing you. He is a good God.

Our other option is to let these events keep us locked in a cycle that devours not only us, but those around us. Putting the past into perspective is to see your suffering through the purposes and hope of God.

Reflections:

On Your Own (5 minutes)

1. Take some time this week to reflect on the Cycle of Abuse. Ask yourself these questions:

- Have you experienced this cycle? How so?
- Do you repeat this cycle with others today when you experience hurt, rejection, or abandonment? How so?
- Have you made a vow in your heart to seek revenge, or vowed that you'll never place yourself in a position to be hurt, rejected, or vulnerable again? If so, how do you live out these inner vows today?
- Are you addicted to any substances or behaviors that developed as a way to numb the painful effects of your losses and/or abuse? What are they, and what benefit do you think they provide?

2. Read Psalms 55 and 56—honest and raw expressions of David in the midst of suffering at the hands of others. Journal what you learn about how to share your suffering with God and about what hope can be found in these psalms.

SESSION 10
THE BROADER SOIL: CULTURE AND PEERS

KEY CONCEPT: The world around us is always communicating ideas, priorities, desires, convictions, values, and beliefs. The *culture* that surrounds us and the *peers* we live alongside are two soil influences through which we receive various messages about how life works. Discerning the difference between the biblically true messages we've absorbed and those that are worldly gives us understanding into how our personal belief systems developed and have been lived out in our relationships and sexuality.

SESSION 10—THE BROADER SOIL: CULTURE AND PEERS

Review and Reflect (15 minutes)

Last Week's Key Concept: When we experience traumatic and painful events such as abuse, loss, and abandonment, we respond and react to a world that is unsafe and unpredictable. As we understand how these profoundly painful experiences have impacted us, and the ways we responded to them, we gain additional insight into how our idolatrous ways of relating to people and life developed. This wisdom guides us in turning from false comforts to the True Comforter, Jesus Christ.

1. What insights did you gain from your personal study of the *Cycle of Abuse*?

2. What did you learn from your study of Psalms 55 and 56? How did you hear your heart as you read how David poured out his?

Exploring a Key Issue (60 minutes)

Read the Key Concept and text aloud and discuss the questions that follow.

Key Concept: The world around us is always communicating ideas, priorities, desires, convictions, values, and beliefs. The *culture* that surrounds us, and the *peers* we live alongside, are two soil influences through which we receive various messages about how life works. Discerning the difference between the biblically true messages we've absorbed and those that are worldly gives us understanding into how our personal belief systems developed and have been lived out in our relationships and sexuality.

From the day we were born, we have been hearing many messages. Through influences such as media, the news, advertising, the classroom, books, television, Internet, etc., as well as our peer relationships, we've absorbed millions of words and ideas. These voices create a surround sound of influence that is constantly speaking, wooing, inviting, negating, and affirming certain beliefs (shoots). Some of these voices have been aligned with the truths of God's Word. Many others, however, have been on a spectrum that at one end is *opposed* to a biblical worldview, while the other end of the spectrum is passionately *antagonistic*. Our relationships, and the way we've understood and expressed our sexuality, are only two of our many personal spheres that bear out the fruit of our belief system.

The Bible doesn't present the world around us (culture, arts, secular thought, etc.) as the ultimate enemy to God and his people. Rather, Scripture tells us plainly, "Finally, be strong in the Lord and in the strength of his might. Put on the whole armor of God, that you may be able to stand against the schemes of the devil. *For we do not wrestle against flesh and blood*, but against the rulers, against the authorities, against the cosmic powers over this present darkness, against the *spiritual forces of evil* in the heavenly places" (Ephesians 6:10–12, emphasis added). This passage tells us that our biggest battle is with the spiritual forces of evil (Satan and the kingdom of darkness), which exerts constant external influence on the world in which we live, and our sinful flesh which exerts influence on the ways we think, feel, and act.

We are not to fear the devil, but we must grow in awareness of how his influence has corrupted the culture in which we have each grown up and in which we presently live. Lies and deceptions, which come at us from numerous influences, blind us to the truth of *who God is, who we are* as daughters of God, and *how we are to live* as sexual and relational beings. Second Corinthians 4:4 says, "the god of this world has blinded the minds of the unbelievers, to keep them from seeing the light of the gospel of the glory of Christ, who is the image of God." Think about what this verse is saying, that Satan *has blinded* the minds of people who exert all sorts of sway through media, entertainment, education, etc.; and we, in turn, are influenced by them! This has deep and wide significance for us as we contemplate how our views of life, sexuality, and relationships may have been watered and nurtured along in their development from a worldly foundation of belief rather than God's truth.

3. Until Jesus Christ returns, the world in which we live will continue to be influenced by our sinful flesh and the "ruler of this world" (John 12:31), who is Satan and who leads the spiritual kingdom of darkness. How have you seen the influence of the domain of darkness in recent years especially in regards to sex and sexuality? What types of stories and themes are "preached" through the world of entertainment? Do you have examples of how your personal convictions regarding sexuality have drifted from a biblical view, in part by the encouragement of cultural voices? If yes, what specific influences contributed to the changes in your convictions?

4. Describe the friends in your life from the following time periods and how you think they influenced you in the ways you understood sex, girls/women, boys/men and what was most important in life: (a) 5–11 years old; (b) 12–18 years old; (c) 19–25 years old.

Read the following and discuss the questions.

God's design for sexuality and the call of Jesus' gospel teach a very different message from what the world—*and our own hearts*—often say. Jesus would have surely used different words and concepts if his desire was to promote me-ism and instant gratification as the norm for his followers. Read just a few quotes from Scripture of what he said, as well as three of his followers: Paul, Peter, and John. These are words spoken to people just like us! The listeners were men and women living in a world full of sensuality, ungodly voices, and temptations to live against God's ways through selfish ambitions and desires.

"If anyone would come after me, let him deny himself and take up his cross daily and follow me."   — Jesus, Luke 9:23

"Now this I say and testify in the Lord, that you must no longer walk as the Gentiles [unbelievers] do, in the futility of their minds. They are darkened in their understanding, alienated from the life of God because of the ignorance that is in them, due to the hardness of their heart. They have become callous and have given themselves up to sensuality, greedy to practice every kind of impurity. But that is not the way you learned Christ!"   — Paul, Ephesians 4:17–20

"Beloved, I urge you as sojourners and exiles to abstain from the passions of the flesh, which wage war against your soul. Keep your conduct among the [unbelieving world] honorable, so that when they speak against you as evildoers, they may see your good deeds and glorify God on the day of visitation."   — Peter, 1 Peter 2:11–12

"Do not love the world or the things in the world. If anyone loves the world, the love of the Father is not in him. For all that is in the world—the desires of the flesh and the desires of the eyes and pride in possessions—is not from the Father but is from the world."
                                        — John, 1 John 2:15–16

The good news of the gospel is that Jesus does not give us commands and then leave us to our own strength, wisdom, and good effort to try to live them out! His commands to die to self, follow after him rather than the world, and to love others pure-heartedly, are actually possible through the power of the Holy Spirit, the very presence of God living within us. The world may speak a robust and convincing message *to us*, but our Lord and Savior dwells *within us*, speaking words of life, hope, and truth.

5. Which of the following passages above most resonate with you as contrary, or opposite, to some of the loudest and most influential peer and

cultural voices in your life? How has a fear of people (not wanting to be left out, craving approval/acceptance, anxious not to be seen as odd or different) fueled some of the sinful choices you've made? Explain your answers.

6. Isaiah 5:20–21 describes the seriousness of using measurements and interpretations of life that are not lined up with God's truth. When we let our lens for life be the beliefs of an ungodly world, an ungodly friend, or our own hearts, which are so prone toward being deceived, we will eventually have a belief system operating within us that is counter to what God says. The fruit of ungodly thinking bears out when we label what is good, evil and what is evil, good; when we call what is bitter, sweet and what is sweet, bitter; when we categorize what is darkness as light, and what is light as darkness. Based on these definitions, we live out our beliefs through our relationships, sexual experiences, and lots of other ways. How are you aware, in your specific areas of relational and sexual sin, that you have called what is bitter, evil, or dark as sweet, good, or light? How have friends influenced you in how you've defined what is good and what is evil, thus encouraging you to pursue certain experiences and to avoid others?

7. It is good to remember once again that soil influences are only that: *influences*! The world around us and even the closest of friends cannot *force or make us* sin. This is both sobering and encouraging when we consider these wonderful promises for those who belong to Christ Jesus, having been born again and indwelt by the Spirit: "His divine power has granted to us all things

that pertain to life and godliness, through the knowledge of him who called us to his own glory and excellence, by which he has granted to us his precious and very great promises, so that through them you may become partakers of the divine nature, having escaped from the corruption that is in the world because of sinful desire" (2 Peter 1:3–4).

How is it sobering to realize that sinful desires lead to corruption, including corrupting influences? How does this passage encourage you as you consider the day in and day out battle that all followers of Jesus face as we live in a world filled with ungodly influences? Are there any specific steps you can take this week to silence ungodly voices via culture?

Making It Personal (10 minutes)

Read the following aloud and spend time in prayer for each other.

The enemies of God are often described as the world, the flesh (our sinful hearts), and the devil. These three realities are opposed to the wisdom, grace, and hope that is ours through Jesus Christ. While we wrestle not "against flesh and blood," but against the spiritual forces of evil, and as we live in a world filled with evil influences, our Rescuer and Redeemer, the Lord God, has transferred us into the kingdom of his beloved son. "He has delivered us from the domain of darkness and transferred us to the kingdom of his beloved Son, in whom we have redemption, the forgiveness of sins" (Colossians 1:13–14). Even as Ephesians 6:12 should soberly remind us that the kingdom of darkness is our daily enemy, Jesus Christ through his death and resurrection has already accomplished the ultimate death blow to this kingdom, as these encouraging words remind us: "This list [in Ephesians 6:12] of *spiritual rulers, authorities and cosmic powers* gives a sobering glimpse into the devil's allies, *the spiritual forces of evil* who are exceedingly powerful in their exercise of cosmic powers over this present darkness. And yet Scripture makes clear that the enemy host is no match for the Lord who has 'disarmed the rulers and authorities and put them to open shame, by triumphing over them in him" (Colossians 2:15; see also Ephesians 1:19–21)."[5]

On Your Own (5 minutes)

1. Read the following prayer, written over 400 years ago, and reflect on how, as we come to the Lord with this kind of heart attitude, the voices in this world that might distract us from Christ grow quiet:

> *Above all things, and in all things, O my soul, rest in the Lord always, for He is the everlasting rest of the saints.*
>
> *Grant me, O loving Jesus, to rest in Thee above every creature (Romans 8:19–22); above all health and beauty, above all glory and honor, above all power and dignity, above all knowledge and subtility, above all riches and arts, above all joy and gladness, above all fame and praise, above all sweetness and comfort, above all hope and promise, above all desert and desire. Above all gifts and favors that Thou canst give and pour upon us, above all mirth and exultation that the mind can receive and feel; finally, all the host of heaven above all finally above angels and archangels, and above all the host of Heaven, above all things visible and invisible, above all that is not Thee, my God.[6]*

2. In the midst of all the struggles and joy we experience on this earth, the Bible consistently encourages us to set our hearts, minds, and hopes on Christ and things above. Thomas à Kempis (the author of the prayer above), understood that he could only truly rest in the Lord Jesus who is our Savior, Friend, Redeemer, and . . . *Home*. Learning to be "at home" with Jesus as we rest and believe in the promises of the gospel will result in a reframing of our unique soil. We can give our soil influences permission to define and govern us, or we can allow them to be a pathway to God. Read Colossians 3:1–4 and journal about the difference it makes, in regards to honestly facing our soil to have our hearts and minds set on things above.

3. Without the truth of God's Word, it would be easy for us to let our earthly experiences be what controls us the most, viewing ourselves and this world as our broken home: unsafe, damaged, and irreparable. Through Jesus we have a *Healing Home* as God our Father forgives us, comes to make *his home **in us***, and takes our heartbreaking experiences to grow us into women who look like Jesus. Session 11 will explore these concepts further as we delve a little bit more into how we've each craved and sought to feel at home through relationships and sexual experiences.

4. Our families are a primary place we begin to learn what it means to be emotionally at home or not. What was the emotional atmosphere of your family/home environment as you grew up? Did it model emotional honesty, or being shut down? Did you feel safe to share hurts, fears, anger, and confusions, or did you feel unsafe and scared to express emotions like this? How were you comforted when you expressed hurt, fear, or sadness? Journal out your thoughts and come prepared to the next session, ready to share your reflections.

SESSION 11
LOOKING FOR YOUR EMOTIONAL
HOME IN ALL THE WRONG PLACES

KEY CONCEPT: Many influences impact our sense of belonging and of feeling secure, valued, known, and loved. When we search outside Jesus and seek to establish these feelings through an "emotional home" in people and/or sexual experiences, the result is idolatry and is disastrous. God's offer of home, unlike people or sex, provides what is *truly* secure, continual, comforting, peaceful, and profoundly intimate.

SESSION 11—LOOKING FOR YOUR EMOTIONAL HOME IN ALL THE WRONG PLACES

Review and Reflect (15 minutes)

Open your session in prayer. Review last week's Key Concept and discuss the questions that follow.

Last Week's Key Concept: The world around us is always communicating ideas, priorities, desires, convictions, values, and beliefs. The *culture* that surrounds us, and the *peers* we live alongside, are two soil influences through which we receive various messages about how life works. Discerning the difference between the biblically true messages we've absorbed and those that are worldly gives us understanding into how our personal belief systems developed and have been lived out in our relationships and sexuality.

1. What encouraged you as you reflected on the prayer by Thomas à Kempis, along with Colossians 3:1–4, in regards to the reality that our truest identity and home is in Jesus? How does it impact you to know that you are "hidden" in Christ (Colossians 3:3)?

2. How would you describe the emotional atmosphere of your home life growing up? What was healthy/helpful? Unhealthy/unhelpful?

Exploring the Key Issue (60 minutes)

Read this week's Key Concept and the section that follows. Then, discuss the questions afterward.

Key Concept: Many influences impact our sense of belonging and of feeling secure, valued, known, and loved. When we search outside Jesus and seek to establish these feelings through an "emotional home" in people and/or sexual experiences, the result is idolatry and is disastrous. God's offer of home, unlike people or sex, provides what is *truly* secure, continual, comforting, peaceful, and profoundly intimate.

How do we learn what to *do* with our emotions? It may seem like an odd question but it's an important one because our creative Creator designed us to feel, to have internal sensations, reactions, and passions. In the Bible we learn that God is a being, not a robot, and that he feels too. Consider Jesus, the *radiance of God's glory and the exact imprint of God's nature* (Hebrews 1:3), who cried, got angry, felt turmoil and anguish, and expressed love, tender care, and affection. We are created in God's image and we bear his image through our entire being including our emotions. We feel lots of things all the time, but the ability to feel and express ourselves freely and without shame was lost when sin entered the world and was replaced by *fear* and *selfishness*. While we live on this earth we will continue to crave emotional peace, comfort, and safety and to hunger for experiences that soothe us and give a sense of being safe and secure emotionally . . . *an emotional home.*

So back to the question of how we each learn what to do with our emotions. There are lots of factors that teach us how to understand and respond to what goes on inside us: God's truth through his Word, significant relationships, the emotional environment in our homes growing up, painful trauma, joyful experiences, and whether the world of people (through our peers and strangers) has felt safe or dangerous are all influences through which we learn:

- How to express what we're feeling in healthy ways, *or to keep troubling emotions buried inside.*
- To feel the weight of painful emotions through our relationship with God and others *or to destructively self-soothe so as to avoid troubling emotions.*

- To receive the Lord's comfort (through his Spirit, Word, and godly relationships) when we ache and hurt *or to run toward broken cisterns that temporarily soothe, or distract, our hurting hearts.*
- To develop patterns of connecting (attaching, bonding) with people in healthy and holy ways, *or clinging to people (and how our relating with them makes us feel) in unhealthy emotional dependence.*
- How to move toward others with loving initiative *or to habitually withdraw and remain emotionally detached.*

An emotional home might be described as a place or relationship where you feel accepted and emotionally safe for who you are and what you feel. Words such as *comfort, connectedness, rest, peace, love, warmth*, and *security* describe it well. When we look away from the Lord Jesus and strive to secure a sense of home through an all-consuming friendship (fueled by a craving to be fully known and to possess) via sexual experiences, being someone's cherished #1 or need-meeter, or being constantly connected/attached to someone, the result *isn't* a healthy emotional home. When we look for home in people and sexual experiences, pushing Jesus to the side, we eventually return to the very things we're running away from and desperately want to avoid: *pain and loneliness.*

3. What is your reaction to these thoughts?

4. How have you learned what to do with emotions? In the list above, which phrases do you most resonate with as you consider your upbringing and as you honestly assess your relational patterns now as an adult?

5. "When we look for 'home' in people and sexual experiences, pushing Jesus to the side, we eventually return to the very things we're running away from and desperately want to avoid: *pain and loneliness.*" Has this been true in your life? How have your sexual partners and/or emotionally entangled/ obsessive relationships given you a sense of home?

Read the following and discuss the questions.

Much of the time, our sexual and relational responses to a broken and painful world are ways we've learned to manage and handle the pain we experience. Many women who began to masturbate as little girls will say they discovered it was an effective way to self-soothe when they felt sad, scared, lonely, or bored. Other women realize that the emotional comfort felt through the sexual attention of others (boys/men, girls/women) becomes an intoxicating way *to feel good.* Other self-comforting strategies may have been food, pornography, sports, self-injury, school, or entertainment. Most of us, when we do not learn as children how to be comforted in healthy ways, will discover our own ways to ease, numb, or distract ourselves from internal turmoil. Adult patterns of sexual sin often have their roots in pain that have not been healed by Jesus and the balm of his Word.

Our hearts, sinful and prone to deception, crave the comfort of what we've thought are emotional homes, but are in reality "broken cisterns." We sinfully turn from the Lord and toward these sources of self-soothing. Sex and/ or unhealthy relating become a compulsive, sinful pattern to soothe and ease the angst of what we're feeling. God's design for all of life is experienced in broken ways by all of us—because we all have sinful hearts! Our sexual sin and our unhealthy relational patterns are cousins to obsessive eating, workaholism, spendaholism, body obsession, drug and alcohol "highs," cutting, and binging, among other self-comforting strategies.

6. What do you think would be initial steps of faith and obedience for you to turn back to the Lord and away from the comfort of sin in your life?

Read the following Scripture passages aloud and discuss the question at the end.

> In you, O LORD, do I take refuge;
>   let me never be put to shame!
> In your righteousness deliver me and rescue me;
>   incline your ear to me, and save me!
> Be to me a rock of refuge,
>   to which I may continually come;
> You have given the command to save me,
>   for you are my rock and my fortress. (Psalm 71:1–3)

> Lord, you have been our dwelling place in all generations.
> Before the mountains were brought forth,
>   or ever you had formed the earth and the world,
>   from everlasting to everlasting you are God. (Psalm 90:1–2)

> Jesus answered him, "If anyone loves me, he will keep my word and my Father will love him and *we will come to him and make our home with him.*" (John 14:23, emphasis added)

God is a trustworthy refuge to which we can continually come because he dwells within his people constantly, permanently, and lovingly. We don't earn this or have to perform to "keep him in our home." Because he is faithful to his promise to remain, by faith we can rest securely in his comfort and peace.

7. How is the home that God offers to us different from what your enmeshed friendships, sexual partnerships, or a fantasy world of your own making have given to you? What does God give to you that sin cannot?

Making It Personal (10 minutes)

Read the following text aloud and close the time in prayer.

Scripture helps us understand how God is compassionately aware of our broken ways of expressing our hearts. Psalm 147:3 says, "He heals the brokenhearted and binds up their wounds." The word *brokenhearted* includes broken emotions. Regardless of how our unhealthy emotional patterns started or how we've watered them with our own selfish choices, God is able to heal and sanctify us. He is tender toward us, as some patterns may have been learned when we were little girls when we didn't know any better. He is also our holy and heart-changing Savior who can free us from our self-serving and ungodly responses to life when it becomes painful, scary, or uncomfortable. This is what Jesus *promised* to do (Isaiah 61:1–3; Luke 4:18–20)!

God's Word clearly reveals that he not only heals our broken hearts but that he has committed to live among and *within* his people. He is home for those who believe in Jesus and abide in him through faith (John 14:23; 15:4–7). God has come to live within his children through the Spirit. He says that *he will make a home in us* (John 14:23) and commands us to live a lifestyle of abiding, making our homes in him and his Word (John 15). This is an intimacy that is spiritual and actual, but also very different from sexual intimacy with a person. Jesus offers us union with himself, literally joining his very being to us within our souls. Godly, emotionally intimate relationships we may have, as well as the godly sexual relating between husbands and wives, are gifts for us and meant to be a signpost to the "at home-ness" which is ours in Christ. If these are new thoughts, perhaps even puzzling or scary to you, that's OK! God wants to teach you his ways and is patient with his children as we come to him with our questions and fears. Just as our unholy and unhealthy patterns grew over time, so also will our faith and confidence in God as our true home grow over time.

For further study regarding how women seek escape from painful emotions, see Appendix D on page 178, *Facing Anger and Emotional Pain*.

On Your Own (5 minutes)

1. Review the following scriptures. As you do so, reflect on how God both *is* our home and has come to make his home *in* us, and how this impacts your own broken patterns of seeking home and comfort through relational and sexual sin. What will be the evidence (fruit!) that God dwells within us?

    a.   Psalm 90:1

    b.   John 14 (all)

    c.   John 15:1–11

    d.   Psalm 71 (all)

2. Session 12 will talk about how our soil is redeemed through the Lord. *To redeem* means to buy back, to return something to its rightful master so that whatever is redeemed can then flourish and be experienced according to its original design. While we live on this earth, we will not experience complete freedom from sin or brokenness in our emotions, relationships, and sexuality. However, considering all the various soil influences discussed so far, journal out how you have experienced God bringing redemption and healing to any of them. For example, what are you learning about broken families and how God can redeem painful or disappointing history we have? Or, in light of painful trauma you may have experienced: How is God taking what Satan wanted to use for evil and using it to grow you in Christlikeness?

3. Hint (!) for number 1 above, one of the "fruits" that will grow in our lives is our prayer relationship with the Lord. He wants us to talk to him about

*every*thing! Spend time this week praying for each of the women in the group, asking God to help them believe he is their safe home, and that each will take obedient steps toward him, and away from sin this week.

SESSION 12
REDEEMING OUR SOIL: KNOWING GOD AS FATHER, HOME, AND COMFORTER

KEY CONCEPT: Soil influences—*experiences we have that arise from living in a broken world and that are outside our control*—are covered under God's promise to redeem us from all lawlessness. This lawlessness includes not only *our* sins, but also sin directly committed against us and the indirect effects of living in a broken and fallen world. God's redeeming love comes to us with grace and mercy and reveals him as the Lord God who is Savior, as well as our true Father, Home, and Comforter. Understanding these characteristics of God—and what they mean concerning our identity in him—helps us live a life of love rather than pursuing sexual sin and idolatrous relationships.

SESSION 12—REDEEMING OUR SOIL: KNOWING GOD AS FATHER, HOME, AND COMFORTER

Review and Reflect (15 minutes)

Open your session in prayer. Review last week's Key Concept, and then discuss the questions that follow.

Last Week's Key Concept: Many influences impact our sense of belonging, having value, and of feeling secure, known, and loved. When we search outside Jesus and seek to establish these feelings through an "emotional home" in people and/or sexual experiences, the result is idolatry and is disastrous. God's offer of home, unlike people or sex, provides what is *truly* secure, continual, comforting, peaceful, and profoundly intimate.

1. What new insights did you gain from your study of the Bible passages regarding God as our home, refuge, and safe place?

2. Which of the sessions regarding soil influences has been most helpful for you? Which was most difficult? Explain your answers.

Exploring the Key Issue (60 minutes)

Read this week's Key Concept and the paragraphs that follow. Then, discuss the questions afterward.

Key Concept: Soil influences—*experiences we have that arise from living in a broken world and that are outside our control*—are covered under God's promise to redeem us from all lawlessness. This lawlessness includes not only *our* sins, but also sin directly committed against us and the indirect effects of living in a broken and fallen world. God's redeeming love comes to us with grace and mercy and reveals him as the Lord God who is Savior, as well as our true Father, Home, and Comforter. Understanding these characteristics of God—and what they mean concerning our identity in him—helps us live a life of love rather than pursuing sexual sin and idolatrous relationships.

> For the grace of God has appeared, bringing salvation for all people, training us to renounce ungodliness and worldly passions, and to live self-controlled, upright and godly lives in the present age, waiting for our blessed hope, the appearing of the glory of our great God and Savior Jesus Christ, who gave himself for us to redeem us from all lawlessness and to purify for himself a people for his own possession who are zealous for good works. (Titus 2:11–14)

> What agreement has the temple of God with idols? For we are the temple of the living God; as God said,
>   "I will make my dwelling among them and walk among them,
>   and I will be their God,
>   and they shall be my people.
> Therefore go out from their midst,
>   and be separate from them, says the Lord,
> and touch no unclean thing;
>   then I will welcome you,
>   and I will be a father to you,
>   and you shall be sons and daughters to me,
>   says the Lord Almighty." (2 Corinthians 6:16–18)

Over the last several sessions, we've delved into a variety of soil influences we may encounter and their potential impact upon us. God's Word instructs us to be courageously honest about life in this fallen world, but he doesn't leave us in our fallenness or our brokenheartedness. He beckons us to come to him for healing from pain, freedom from enslaving patterns of sin, and wisdom to understand his transforming truth. As mentioned already, soil influences are just that—*influences*, not identities. God, as Father, Home, and Comforter, identifies himself and us in ways that help us to understand how he redeems our soil experiences.

3. Review the two Bible passages above. What do they say about God and about his promises for those who are his sons and daughters? What are God's commands for those who are his?

4. How can the promise of God's loving fatherhood and his call for us to lives of love and holy zeal change the way you view your family of origin? How do you need God to change the focus of your zeal? Quietly write your private reflections below.

Read the following aloud, then discuss the questions that follow:

Jesus promised in John 14:23 that he and his father would come to make their home in those who love him. Likewise, 2 Corinthians 6:16–18 quotes the Old Testament in describing how God would dwell or walk among his people (Leviticus 26:12). Now that Jesus has come and sent the Spirit, God actually dwells *within* his people! This is what Jesus' teaching in John 15 describes, using the analogy of branches abiding, remaining, and *making a home* in the vine. We are the branches and Jesus is the vine. As the true vine, Jesus gives us spiritual life, safety, security, and a resting place. He is our true home!

5. In Session 11, we discussed how women often crave and seek to secure an emotional home in people through idolatrous dependency and/or sex. How

can a deeper understanding and trust in Jesus as your true home change the way you view people, sex, and relationships?

6. Consider again Jesus' analogy in John 15, as he called himself the vine and us his branches. Using your imagination, what do you think holy relating would look like between the branches and the vine? List your thoughts below and then share with the group.

7. What are you most fearful of as you contemplate God's command to abide in him and his word alone, rather than seeking a "home" in a person? Write out your private thoughts below.

Finally, consider again the rich promises of 2 Corinthians 1:3–4: "Blessed be the God and Father of our Lord Jesus Christ, the Father of mercies and God of all comfort, who comforts us in all our affliction, so that we may be able to comfort those who are in any affliction, with the comfort with which we ourselves are comforted by God."

Our God is a Father of *mercies*, which means he is tender and compassionate to us as we experience the misery of sin. Our God is also *the* God of *all* comfort, and *all means all!* We receive his comfort by faith, which is radically different from the comfort we may experience through sex with a man, woman, or ourselves. Physical and emotional comfort that comes via people and sexual experiences may temporarily soothe our hearts, but will not last. It cannot, for these experiences do not have the power to enter into our beings as Christ does! He alone, as our home, dwells within, providing lasting, soul-healing comfort for his people. Growth in holy relationships will be a fruit for each of us as we learn to bring our relational pain to Christ and receive his comfort, rather than seeking it through our sin.

8. How are you learning that, as you look to Christ for comfort, his comfort goes deeper into your heart and brings peace, even when he does not give the emotional or sexual payback of sin? Share with the group a recent experience in which the comfort of God was real to your heart, even as the circumstances in your life may have been painful, hard, or scary.

Making It Personal (10 minutes)

Read the following aloud:

> You have taken from me my closest friends
>   and have made me repulsive to them.
> I am confined and cannot escape;
>   my eyes are dim with grief.
> I call to you, O LORD, every day;
>   I spread out my hands to you. (Psalm 88:8–9 NIV)

> There is a way that seems right to a man,
>   but its end is the way to death.
> Even in laughter the heart may ache,
>   and the end of joy may be grief. (Proverbs 14:12–13)

The writer of Psalm 88 anguishes over the loss of friendship due to abandonment and rejection and calls out to God in the midst of his pain. In Proverbs, Solomon wisely describes how the human condition is woven with both happiness and heartache, with joy and with the grief that comes from loss, disappointment, and struggle. But as we've learned, God does not leave us alone in our losses. He comes to us in his Son, Jesus Christ, spoken of in Isaiah 53:3–4a as the one who, "was despised and rejected by men; a man of sorrows, and acquainted with grief; and as one from whom men hide their faces he was despised, and we esteemed him not. Surely he has borne our griefs and carried our sorrows."

Take turns reading 2 Corinthians 1:3–4; Titus 2:11–14; and John 15:4–8. Then close your time together as a group, praying through one of the themes included in these passages.

On Your Own (5 minutes)

Read the following, and answer the reflective questions in preparation for the next session.

God invites us to come to him and lay bare our feelings of loss, hurt, disappointment, abandonment, rejection, and desires for connection and intimacy that were never fulfilled. He receives us with mercy and comforts us in our grief. Scripture helps us to fully express our emotions to the Lord as we see this modeled in the Psalms, and to be truthful about how we've denied the hurt we've experienced. As we honestly face our emotions, we can also grow in acknowledging how we've turned to people, sex, or addictive substances— living a life of craving to meet our own desires and feel satisfied.

1. Read Romans 13:8–14. What kinds of "loss" happen when we make no provision for the flesh and instead commit to put on the Lord Jesus Christ? In other words, what will it cost you to follow Jesus fully? What will you need to let go of, and how much do you think it will hurt to do so?

2. Take time to sit in the presence of the Lord with your grief, and allow the feelings of loss to be felt and processed, so that you may experience true comfort. Then, read the story of Jesus in the Garden of Gethsemane in Matthew 26:36–46. What do you learn from Jesus about responding to grief, abandonment, disappointment, fear, and loneliness?

SESSION 13
THE ROOTS: OUR DESIRES

KEY CONCEPT: Our desires are what motivate us. What we do with those desires can either be the expression of a Christ-worshipping heart or a creation-worshipping heart. They can be good or evil, depending on the motivation behind them. Understanding what desires tend to rule us in selfish ways helps us unpack our understanding of the development of our sinful behaviors.

SESSION 13—THE ROOTS: OUR DESIRES

Review and Reflect (15 minutes)

Open your session in prayer. Review last week's Key Concept, and then discuss the questions that follow.

Last Week's Key Concept: Soil influences—*experiences we have that arise from living in a broken world and that are outside our control*—are covered under God's promise to redeem us from all lawlessness. This lawlessness includes not only *our* sins, but also sin directly committed against us and the indirect effects of living in a broken and fallen world. God's redeeming love comes to us with grace and mercy and reveals him as the Lord God who is Savior, as well as our true Father, Home, and Comforter. Understanding these characteristics of God—and what they mean concerning our identity in him—helps us live a life of love rather than pursuing sexual sin and idolatrous relationships.

1. What did you learn from studying Romans 13:8–14 and considering the kinds of loss we encounter as we make no provision for the flesh and instead put on Jesus?

2. How did the account of Jesus in the Garden of Gethsemane encourage you? What did you learn from Jesus' example about responding to grief, abandonment, disappointment, fear, and loneliness?

Exploring the Key Issue (60 minutes)

Read this week's Key Concept and the section that follows. Then, discuss the questions afterward.

Key Concept: Our desires are what motivate us. What we do with those desires can either be the expression of a Christ-worshipping heart or a creation-worshipping heart. They can be good or evil, depending on the motivation behind them. Understanding what desires tend to rule us in selfish ways helps us unpack our understanding of the development of our sinful behaviors.

This session addresses the next component of the Tree Model—*the roots*. Roots refer to our God-given desires for relationship, intimacy, and significance, which can become bent toward seeking satisfaction in self-oriented ways. The Bible calls this pursuit of self "idolatry." Idolatry originates from a selfish sinful heart that craves satisfaction in ways outside God's design. One woman desires to be loved and cherished, and therefore seeks sexual attention from a man because it makes her feel loved. Another becomes enmeshed emotionally and sexually with another woman because it feels comforting and secure to be someone's #1. Another woman watches porn and escapes to a fantasy world of her own making because it's a world of relationships in which she's the center and always gets what she wants. Common desires—for love, intimacy, security, safety, power, status, approval, belonging, comfort, significance, and affirmation—can quickly grow into selfish demands, thus bearing the fruit of sexual sin.

"His divine power has granted to us all things that pertain to life and godliness, through the knowledge of him who called us to his own glory and excellence, by which he has granted to us his precious and very great promises, so that through them you may become partakers of the divine nature, having escaped from the corruption that is in the world because of *sinful desire*" (2 Peter 1:3–4, emphasis added).

3. What desires have motivated you in your sexual sin, or idolatrous relationships?

4. Are desires ever good? Can they be holy? Explain.

5. Review the chart below together as a group. Which desires seem to easily hijack your heart? How has this motivated your pursuit of your personal idols? Share specific examples or stories, if possible.

How Does a Desire Become an Idol?

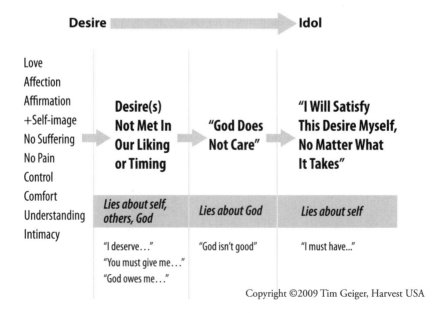

Desire		→	Idol

Love Affection Affirmation +Self-image No Suffering No Pain Control Comfort Understanding Intimacy	**Desire(s) Not Met In Our Liking or Timing**	**"God Does Not Care"**	**"I Will Satisfy This Desire Myself, No Matter What It Takes"**
	Lies about self, others, God	*Lies about God*	*Lies about self*
	"I deserve…" "You must give me…" "God owes me…"	"God isn't good"	"I must have…"

Copyright ©2009 Tim Geiger, Harvest USA

Making It Personal (10 minutes)

Read 2 Peter 1:3–8 together as a group, and then read the paragraph below:

We can grow in being women who desire faithfulness, virtue, knowledge, self-control, steadfastness, godliness, brotherly (and sisterly!) affection, and love. In addition, through Christ we can grow into women who *have* these qualities. Our desires *can change* through the power of the gospel. As our hearts slowly change over time, we desire the Lord more than we desire sin and the fruits of sin. Christian faith leads us not to a list of rules or steps but to a person, Jesus Christ, who changes us from the inside out!

Spend time in prayer as a group, asking God to grow your group members into women whose desires are increasingly surrendered to Jesus, exhibiting the qualities displayed in 2 Peter 1.

On Your Own (5 minutes)

1. Consider these following quotes and answer the question that follows.

"Idols aren't just stone statues. No, idols are the thoughts, desires, longings, and expectations that we worship in the place of the true God. Idols cause us to ignore the true God in search of what we think we need."[7]

"Embracing Christ's beauty and glory is essential [in our battle against sin and idolatry], because worship is a product of love. As the Holy Spirit illumines your heart to Christ's beauty, your love will grow. The false gods that entice will lose their appeal. . . . The sin of unbelief lies at the heart of all other sins and particularly at the heart of idolatry."[8]

How do you think misplaced worship and idolatrous desires have combined together in your own sexual and/or relational sin patterns?

2. Read and reflect on James 1:12–18. How does this passage relate to your personal experience of desires hijacking your heart and motivating you to make sinful choices?

SESSION 14
THE SHOOTS: OUR INTERPRETATIONS AND BELIEFS ABOUT LIFE

KEY CONCEPT: It's been said that children are great observers of life but poor interpreters. We form beliefs and views of life and, based on that, decide how life works. We behave the way we do because of what we believe regarding ourselves, sex, women, men, God, friendships, pain, comfort, pleasure, etc. Often our spoken faith is radically different from our actual lived-out faith. As we grow in understanding and believing God's wisdom and ways, we're able to take steps of faith based on truth rather than lies. Over time faith, love, and obedience will replace the lies we've believed and the former sinful choices we've made.

SESSION 14—THE SHOOTS: OUR INTERPRETATIONS AND BELIEFS ABOUT LIFE

Review and Reflect (15 minutes)

Open in prayer. Read last week's Key Concept aloud, and then discuss the questions that follow.

Last Week's Key Concept: Our desires are what motivate us. What we do with those desires can either be the expression of a Christ-worshipping heart or a creation-worshipping heart. They can be good or evil, depending on the motivation behind them. Understanding what desires tend to rule us in selfish ways helps us unpack our understanding of the development of our sinful behaviors.

1. What role do you think misplaced worship and idolatrous desires have played in your sexual and/or relational sin patterns? How has your sin soothed desires that the Lord hasn't satisfied in the way *you* wanted?

2. What did you learn from your reflection upon James 1:12–18? In what ways have your desires led you into sin?

Exploring the Key Issue (60 minutes)

Read the Key Concept and the section that follows aloud. Then, discuss the questions afterward.

Key Concept: It's been said that children are great observers of life but poor interpreters. We form beliefs and views of life and, based on that, decide how life works. We behave the way we do because of what we believe regarding ourselves, sex, women, men, God, friendships, pain, comfort, pleasure, etc. Often our spoken faith is radically different from our actual lived-out faith. As we grow in understanding and believing God's wisdom and ways, we're able to take steps of faith based on truth rather than lies. Over time faith, love, and obedience will replace the lies we've believed and the former sinful choices we've made.

This session brings us to our last component of the Tree Model—the shoots. The shoots of the tree are the conclusions or worldviews we've developed over the years. Think of the shoots as the lenses through which we view and interpret our world—how we believe "life works." Our interpretations, however, are always tainted by self. We live, relate, respond, and behave out of our faulty understandings of God, men, women, relationships, sex, gender, etc. Thus, we need to develop transformed minds that reflect God's truth. This is how Romans 12:2 describes it (emphasis added): "Do not be conformed to this world, but be transformed by *the renewal of your mind*, that by testing you may discern what is the will of God, what is good and acceptable and perfect."

3. What shoots are you aware of that have fueled your sexual behavior with men and/or women? In other words, what do you seek *to get* and what do you seek *to avoid* through your sexual behaviors?

4. Chris Thurman says, "Your brain is a tape deck. It can both record and play back, and it has access to a personal library of thousands of tapes ready to play at a moment's notice. These tapes hold all the beliefs, attitudes, and

expectations that you have 'recorded' during your life."[9] What's your reaction to this quote? What tapes do you tend to replay in your mind, and why? What memories of events or incidents from earlier in your life seem to start the tape?

5. Read Romans 8:5–9 aloud. What encouragements and warnings do you find in these verses? Which resonate with you most right now?

6. What steps can you take so that your self-centered or self-deceiving shoots can be transformed into godly, truth-based worldviews? What keeps you from taking these steps?

Making It Personal (10 minutes)

Read the following, and spend time in prayer together.

Our worldview can be described as our attitudes and beliefs—the conclusions we've reached based upon our shaping influences and life experiences. We formulated a set of beliefs about life as we grew up, and we continue to live out of those beliefs. We must see and expose where these beliefs do not align with the truth of Scripture. Only a worldview derived from Scripture offers hope and a pair of eyeglasses that are "clear."

Does it feel overwhelming to consider changing your belief systems? To take steps to have your mind set on the Spirit rather than on your own desires, understandings, and perhaps false interpretations?

The good news is it's not all up to us. *Jesus* has come to set the captive free (Luke 4:18–19). Our thoughts can be imprisoned and held captive to lies, the pains of our past, and selfishness. Thankfully, the freeing power of Jesus reaches even to our thought lives! Second Corinthians 10:5 tells us to take every thought captive to Christ, and God doesn't command us to do things that are impossible! True, in our own power they can't be done, but through the Spirit of Christ within us we can have transformed minds and "shoots"!

On Your Own (5 minutes)

This week the homework includes a lot of reading. Take the time to read through Appendix E, "Common Lies" (p. 187), and answer the reflective questions below. As you read, reflect not only on the lies, but the truths from God's Word. There are many Scripture references to read as you have time, but be sure to read them over the course of this week! Come to the next session prepared to share your insights.

1. What lies do you believe about God and your sin, and why? Which Scriptures most encouraged you, in light of this?

2. What lies do you believe about *yourself and others*? Where did you get these lies, and whom did you learn them from? Write down your answers, and how those lies were watered and nurtured in your life so that you grew to own them.

3. What connections do you see between the lies you believe and your sinful behaviors and inclinations?

SESSION 15
THE SHOOTS: WHAT WE BELIEVE ABOUT GENDER

KEY CONCEPT: What does it mean to you to be a woman, and is it good? What does it mean to express oneself in a feminine manner? To *be* feminine? How are we to view men and maleness? Culture and pop psychology give their opinions and ideas—and true to form, those opinions have changed and morphed throughout history. God's Word clearly says that God created people as male and female (Genesis 1:27). The ravages of the fall have impacted each person, even at the level of our gender. No one experiences their femaleness or maleness without feeling the impact of this brokenness.

SESSION 15—THE SHOOTS: WHAT WE BELIEVE ABOUT GENDER

Review and Reflect (15 minutes)

Open in prayer. Read last week's Key Concept aloud, and then discuss the questions that follow.

Last Week's Key Concept: It's been said that children are great observers of life but poor interpreters. We form beliefs and views of life and, based on that, decide how life works. We behave the way we do because of what we believe regarding ourselves, sex, women, men, God, friendships, pain, comfort, pleasure, etc. Often our spoken faith is radically different from our actual lived-out faith. As we grow in understanding and believe God's wisdom and ways, we're able to take steps of faith based on truth rather than lies. Over time faith, love, and obedience will replace the lies we've believed and the former sinful choices we've made.

1. After reading the list of "Common Lies" (p. 187), which lies about God did you find yourself connecting with most? Explain.

2. What lies have you believed about yourself and others? As best you can determine, how did those lies come about? How does God's Word counter these lies and help you see the truth more clearly?

3. How has God encouraged you this week, as you've reflected on the possibility of having a transformed mind?

Exploring the Key Issue (60 minutes)

Read the Key Concept and the section that follows aloud. Then, discuss the questions afterward.

Key Concept: What does it mean to you to be a woman, and is it good? What does it mean to express oneself in a feminine manner? To *be* feminine? How are we to view men and maleness? Culture and pop psychology give their opinions and ideas—and true to form, those opinions have changed and morphed throughout history. God's Word clearly says that God created people as male and female (Genesis 1:27). The ravages of the fall have impacted each person, even at the level of our gender. No one experiences their femaleness or maleness without feeling the impact of this brokenness.

Gender identity is an aspect of ourselves we often ignore or push under the rug. But because God made people male or female, we must seek to understand gender from a biblical lens. Some of us grew up not feeling truly female, as if we were in some neuter or "asexual" category. Others of us disdained our femaleness and craved being male instead. Still others may have enjoyed being female, but not necessarily for God-honoring reasons (i.e., because of what we could get from men and/or women).

We must take a step back and examine honestly what we think and feel about being women. God did not make a mistake in making us female, but had good and loving purposes in his creation of women as female image-bearers. Grasping a biblical view of gender will help us discern how we may have bought into the culture's increasingly confused definition of gender, and how that has impacted the way we think and feel about being female.

A biblical view of gender also helps us grow in how we view men. In their maleness, men reflect God's image differently than women do, and neither image is more worthy or precious in God's eyes. It's important to understand how sin has not only distorted our views of being female, but also our views of who God created men to be. God's Word brings clarity to the confusion.

4. When you hear the words *woman*, *female*, and *girl*, what are the first words that come to mind for each? Why do you think *those* words, in particular?

5. Has your experience been that of feeling different or "other" from other girls, or that being female was something you wanted to draw attention to? Regardless of your answer, explain.

6. Bearing in mind your primary area of struggle, consider the following questions:
- If you're same-sex attracted: When were you first aware of being attracted to other girls—when you began to believe the "shoot" that emotional and sexual connection with women equals life?
- If you've sought life and value through sexual encounters with men: When did you begin to believe the "shoot" that emotional and sexual intimacy with men equals life?
- If your struggle has been with pornography and masturbation: How has this impacted your views of being a woman?

7. Do you cover, avoid, and/or reject "looking" female or what you think feminine looks like? Or do you dress provocatively, drawing attention to certain parts of your body? Either way, what are the shoots that fuel your personal style? What do you seek to gain or avoid by the way you present yourself?

8. Jesus—God and man—loved, honored, befriended, healed, served, and was served by . . . women! What are examples from his life that prove he believed women were worthy of honor, respect, and care?

Making It Personal (10 minutes)

Being created by God as a woman is part of our identity. Many of us remain disconnected emotionally and mentally from this part of our identity, and yet a significant part of our healing must touch this aspect of who we are. Becoming a whole person means becoming a whole woman, embracing the fact that we were chosen by God to be women, and accepting and cherishing our own unique femaleness. Further, healing must touch how we see other women so that we begin choosing to embrace the "world of women" in new and redemptive ways.

For additional study, there are many articles and resources on the website of the Council for Biblical Manhood and Womanhood, www.cbmw.org. A biblical view of gender leads us to consider how God designed us both as image-bearers, but that we bear his image differently in our femaleness, than men do in being male. Many of the "defining characteristics" of women that we've been presented have been largely based on personality traits and interests, which can be different for different women. Some of us fit these characteristics fairly well, while others of us do not—either naturally or willfully. But ultimately, we find our true feminine purpose in the partnership with our brothers that God set up in the beginning, to work together as spiritual family in discipling spiritual image-bearers of God and to bring order to the created world (Genesis 1:27–28).

On Your Own (5 minutes)

Gender is included in the truth of Colossians 1:16: "All things were created through [Jesus] and for [Jesus]." This includes the male image as expressed in men. This week's homework will guide you to honestly consider how you view men and maleness. Read the passage below, and work through the reflective questions that accompany each section, in preparation for the next session.

Men, Maleness, and the Redemption of Jesus

In this fallen world, broken men express their broken sexuality against women, and some women have experienced this in traumatic ways. However, this doesn't discount the goodness of God's design of men, and the gospel reality that God is redeeming broken manhood and distortions of godly masculinity—just as he is redeeming broken womanhood and distortions of godly femininity. Romans 12:1–2 instructs us not only to have a transformed view of ourselves, but also of men (and all aspects of life). We're not to be conformed to the world's way of interpretation based *on self*. The process of transformation *is* possible as we allow our minds to be gradually aligned to God's gospel of grace, healing, forgiveness, love, hope, and trust. His gospel compels us to consistently live out our faith "horizontally" and "vertically" at the same time. Our relationship to God impacts our relationships with people. The way we love—*and don't love*—people impacts how we relate to God. See 1 John 5:1–3, for just one passage that ties these realities together.

1. When you hear the words *man, male,* and *boy,* what first comes to mind for each word? To what degree do you think your views of men are based on cultural assumptions, stereotypes, or personal experiences? List the stereotypes you believe about men.

Colossians 1:13–17 explains that all things (including men) are created *through* Jesus and *for* Jesus. Broken men express their own broken sexuality, and many women have experienced this in traumatic ways. However, this doesn't discount the goodness of God's creation, which sinful and selfish men and women have polluted.

Sadly, many of us have had negative experiences with men, on a broad continuum ranging from annoying to abusive. Some of these experiences have been traumatic in significant, life-impacting ways. Yet men are redeemable, even as we are. And sin done against us can also be redeemed by the Lord. It's crucial that we all honestly face the internal anger, hurt, fear, and confusion that are connected to our experiences with men. This is a process that God leads us through. As he does so, he provides grace, courage, and comfort. One of the glories of God's work of redemption is that, while it doesn't undo past sin and hurt, it does bring healing of brokenheartedness.

2. Read Isaiah 61:1–4. Reflect specifically on how the promises of this passage can give you hope in light of traumatic experiences that have come through men. Journal or list out your insights.

Another important step in our freedom and growth is to unpack how we project our views of men onto God, and onto the male image he has created (Genesis 1:27). Male is good, as female is good; however, both genders are in a fallen state this side of heaven. The promise of the gospel is that in and through Christ, both genders can be redeemed so that God is glorified by the way we experience our femaleness and by the way we view men.

Men are a part of God's world and thus our world, too—whether we've enjoyed, ignored, used, or disdained them. We're called to live at peace with others and to regard no one from a worldly point of view (2 Corinthians 5:16–17). However, our painful relationships with men have profoundly contributed to feelings of deep-seated anger and resentment toward them. We must face this anger, bitterness, hurt, and resentment. Step by step, we must allow the Lord to create a new lens through which we view not only men, but our experiences with them. God says, "Fear not, for I am with you; be not dismayed, for I am your God; I will strengthen you, I will help you, I will uphold you with my righteous right hand" (Isaiah 41:10). These are promises to hold on to as we learn to extend the love of Christ toward men. They are our neighbors, and we're called to love our neighbors as ourselves.

3. What do you like or see as positives about men? How have any men in your life exhibited kindness, gentleness, respect, strength, leadership, care, and/or protection toward you? Explain.

4. Read Luke 7–13 with two questions in mind: (a) What do you observe about Jesus as a man relating to needy and hurting people? (b) How do you relate to the women with whom Jesus interacts in these chapters?

Our views of men *can be transformed* as we understand not only the godly manhood of Jesus, but also his ministry to heal, forgive, redeem, and change broken men into godly men. Healthy and holy relating to men comes as our hearts are rewired and our thoughts transformed by God's Word. God enables us to see men rightly—neither disdaining them, nor using them for selfish purposes. The gospel of grace gently grows us to see men as brothers in Christ, needy of him in the same ways we are, *and* as beloved sons of God for whom Jesus died.

5. Ask God to give you insight into your views of men and how your views do or don't align with a biblical perspective.

SESSION 16
UNDERSTANDING THE NATURE OF
HABITUAL SIN PATTERNS

KEY CONCEPT: Life-dominating sin patterns don't form overnight, and sexual addiction and entrenched patterns of relating are no different. Repeated actions become habits over time. As we've explored in earlier lessons, our actions are the expression of our hearts. Our hearts flow toward enslaving, habitual sin patterns, or toward an emerging pattern of life that is increasingly free, holy, and Christlike.

SESSION 16—UNDERSTANDING THE NATURE OF HABITUAL SIN PATTERNS

Review and Reflect (15 minutes)

Open in prayer. Read last week's Key Concept aloud, and then discuss the questions that follow.

Last Week's Key Concept: What does it mean to you to be a woman, and is it good? What does it mean to express oneself in a feminine manner? To *be* feminine? How are we to view men and maleness? Culture and pop psychology give their opinions and ideas—and true to form, those opinions have changed and morphed throughout history. God's Word clearly says that God created people as male and female (Genesis 1:27). The ravages of the fall have impacted each person, even at the level of our gender. No one experiences their femaleness or maleness without feeling the impact of this brokenness.

1. What insights did you gain from your readings and from the reflection questions regarding men and maleness?

2. How do you need healing and courage in order to relate to men as beloved sons of God, created in his image?

3. Now that all of the components of the Tree Model have been addressed, take a glance back at the picture on p. 14. Do you have any questions about

any of the components—heart/seed, soil/influences, roots/desires, shoots/worldviews, or fruit/behaviors?

Exploring the Key Issue (60 minutes)

Read the Key Concept and the section that follows aloud. Then, discuss the questions afterward.

Key Concept: Life-dominating sin patterns don't form overnight, and sexual addiction and entrenched patterns of relating are no different. Repeated actions become habits over time. As we've explored in earlier lessons, our actions are the expression of our hearts. Our hearts flow toward enslaving, habitual sin patterns, or toward an emerging pattern of life that is increasingly free, holy, and Christlike.

From a biblical view, addictions are life-dominating sins or unholy and enslaving habits. They're patterns of behaving and responding that give us the illusion of control over the chaos and pain of our lives, but in the end enslave us rather than give us peace, security, or lasting comfort. All of us battle with the temptation to respond to life from a me-first perspective rather than from a Christ-dependent heart. We all go astray, wandering from the living water of Christ for a variety of reasons. The common denominator for every single human being is that we have a mini-kingdom within us ruled by self, which does not naturally gravitate toward leaning on God's wisdom for navigating a broken world (Proverbs 3:5–7). Habitual patterns of sin are actually self-constructed methods of making our mini-kingdoms work. We self-soothe, numb, or distract ourselves as a way to avoid the discomforts and trials of life—rather than turn to the true king, Jesus.

Although it's not normally thought of as a chemical addiction, that's what sex addiction is, even if indirectly so. Those with sexual and/or relational addictions aren't popping pills, but their addictive behaviors do have a physiological impact. Their bodily sensations trigger responses within the brain via thoughts, actions, and words. The sex-addicted or emotionally addicted/dependent person experiences a state of numbness (from unwanted pain) or euphoria through her behaviors. The habit or addiction grows into an entrenched pattern as this state is achieved over and over, and the craving to return to that state becomes an enslaving pattern. This in no way puts the blame for our sin on our bodies or brains, but serves to show us once again how our entire beings have been impacted by sin. Paul says in 1 Thessalonians 5:23 (emphasis added), "Now may the God of peace himself sanctify you completely, and may your *whole spirit and soul and body* be kept blameless at the coming of our Lord Jesus Christ."

4. What's your response to the above paragraphs? Do you think you're an addict? Explain.

5. How might it be helpful to view your area of sin struggle as a *habitual pattern of sin* rather than merely calling it an addiction?

Take turns reading through the following section aloud, and then discuss the question that follows:

Psychologist Dr. Patrick Carnes developed a model that describes the development of sexual addiction.[10] This model can help us understand how *any* addictive struggle or sin cycle develops, as well as provide an understanding of how freedom and change from sinful patterns can happen.

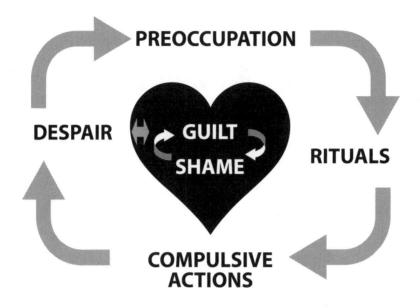

Triggers. In Carnes's model, the trigger is what leads someone into Preoccupation, the first stage of the addictive cycle. Everyone has triggers—physical and/or emotional states that weaken our ability to fight temptation. Common triggers are known by the acronym HALT (hungry, angry, lonely, tired). Other triggers mentioned by women battling habitual relational and sexual sins include boredom, fear, and emotional pain. Triggers can lean us in the direction of sin as our thoughts become preoccupied with what our hearts are craving, or they can lead us to cry out to God for help. Consider the many psalms of David where fear, rejection, attack, and loneliness lead him to God instead of to sin. (Read Psalms 56, 57, and 142 on your own, as examples).

Preoccupation. These behaviors include obsessive thinking, fantasy, and mental euphoric recall, and are the first steps to "opening the door" to a habitual pattern of response. Preoccupation begins to stimulate the brain chemicals that give one a "mood-altering hit." In terms of sexual and relational addictions, preoccupation focuses the mind to think of nothing else but specific sexual and/or emotional experiences or a certain person's response to, or pursuit of, us. The mind wanders to fantasy—a picture, a scenario, a person—with the goal being the feeling of sexual release or emotional comfort. It is also in this initial stage of the cycle that self-deceit enters in, particularly through minimizing or finding excuses for why what you're doing is fine. (e.g., "I'm not hurting anyone," "I can stop any time," or "This is totally normal.")

Ritualization. This is defined as the preparation to act upon desires and pursue the sinful behavior, no matter what the cost. These actions lay the smooth asphalt down, so the path to action is clear and ready to drive on. Another way to describe it is "flirting" with sex or an unhealthy relationship. Typically, this process is so automatic that we don't even recognize it. It begins by intensely pursuing or avoiding people or particular situations. We may begin to isolate or withdraw into silence. We begin to swallow the lie that says we'll find relief, satisfaction, peace, or comfort by acting on the object of our preoccupation. We feel ourselves "come alive" inside. Once the rituals begin, it may feel like you're on auto-pilot, or as if you're watching yourself board this all-too-familiar train and you feel as if you can't get off. The reality, however, is that our eyes and ears are becoming closed to truth and the voice of the Holy Spirit.

Compulsive Actions. This is the acting-out of the sinful behavior. Many women lack awareness of the steps they're taking toward sin. In fact, it often isn't until the point of sexual sin actually happening that awareness of a problem is even on the radar. However, sexual behavior never happens in a vacuum. There is a process leading up to the sexual activity, and thus an identifiable pattern to untangle. The compulsive action or "fix" that gives a sense of comfort, satisfaction, or being loved doesn't last long.

Despair. With the realization of having given in again, feelings of despair set in. The aftereffects begin to flood in—feelings of failure, hopelessness, and "stuckness"; saying to yourself, "I've done it again. I vowed I wouldn't and I've done it again." Life feels unmanageable, and failure triggers and reinforces those feelings that life is out of control and that there's no hope that things can be different.

Guilt and Shame. Feelings of guilt wash over us. "I've done it again. I am a bad and evil person; I deserve whatever bad happens in my life. I feel condemned by God and my own conscience. I deserve wrath, consequences, and punishment." Shame is a close relative to guilt. Guilt is failing standards or expectations outside oneself (such as God's); shame is failing our own standards or expectations. Often during this stage we further our isolation from others; and in doing so, we further increase our feelings of loneliness.

We tell ourselves that if anyone knew the truth they'd freak out and reject us. Hiding is paramount: "I must keep this to myself . . . I can handle it . . . just me and God."

Guilt and shame feed on one another. Together, they produce more despair, isolation, and autonomy, which in turn open the door to greater opportunities to reenter the world of preoccupation/fantasy, ritualization, acting out, etc. The cycle starts all over again.

The *law of diminishing returns* applies here. A greater fix, or more intense experience of the sin, is needed to satisfy the cravings for comfort and escape. There is a continual lust for more as the pain, loneliness, boredom, stress, disappointment, powerlessness, and emptiness need a greater fix to get the same high next time.

6. What can you identify as the common triggers that send you on the path to giving way to sin? Share an experience that illustrates how your triggers work in regard to your habitual sin patterns.

7. Have you experienced escape from temptation at the point of being triggered, as promised in 1 Corinthians 10:13? If so, what happened?

Making It Personal (10 minutes)

Read the following aloud:

Freedom from patterns of sin is possible through Jesus Christ. Nonetheless, we will face the battle against temptation for the rest of our lives. There is hope in realizing that it's normal to struggle. Growth comes as we learn to "struggle well" in the direction of obedience and faith.

Spend time in prayer for each other, focusing your prayers on this passage of Scripture:

> "May God himself, the God of peace, sanctify you through and through. May your whole spirit, soul and body be kept blameless at the coming of our Lord Jesus Christ. *The one who calls you is faithful, and he will do it"* (1 Thessalonians 5:23–24 NIV, emphasis added).

On Your Own (5 minutes)

1. Take time this week to journal and pray about the things you've learned regarding your own battle against habitual sins. Write out a prayer that expresses your hope, angst, weariness, joy, or comfort in your own journey to become a woman more and more free of habitual sins, and increasingly given over to the reign of Jesus—the One who sets captive women free from entangling relationships, life-dominating sexual sins, and disordered desires.

2. Reflect on and journal about any successes or victories you've experienced over your temptations and sin struggles. How has Jesus' influence or power given you steps of victory such as quicker awareness of being tempted, quicker willingness to confess to someone that you gave in, longer periods of time between giving in, etc.? Addictions develop over time *without* a lot of self-awareness of what's happening. Victory over sin, and the formation of new habits, will also form over time, step by step—but *with a focus on being self-aware* of the process of sowing to the Spirit rather than to the flesh (see Galatians 6:7–9).

3. Read again through the description of Carnes's model, which describes the Cycle of Sexual Addiction. List or journal how you see your own patterns

of sin in each of the stages of *Preoccupation, Ritualization, Compulsive Actions,* and *Despair.* As you do so, also think about this: What "shoot issues" have been most influential to your vulnerability to sexual addiction, and any other unwanted and/or sinful sexual or relational patterns? For example, if boredom or loneliness is a trigger toward masturbation, this might reveal a worldview that believes emotional discomfort is to be avoided at all costs. Or if the fear of displeasing someone is a trigger toward obsessive connection with someone, this might reveal a worldview that says the acceptance of people is needed for my emotional survival.

4. Read the section below, ""Two Sides of Change." Journal or list how God's grace and your obedience work together to produce change in your life.

Two Sides of Change

Scripture speaks with clarity about the human heart. It's what is in our heart that directs or controls our behavior—leading us either to enslaving, habitual patterns of sin or to emerging and free patterns of life that are increasingly holy. Earlier lessons explained that the fruit of our lives is a manifestation of either a self-serving heart or a God-worshipping heart. The me-first-oriented heart fosters a habitual pattern of sin and addiction. The God-worshipping heart is a foundation that fosters freedom and a growing desire to live and love others with new strength and purpose.

Our lives have become self-focused, self-sufficient, self-deceiving, self-protective, self-contemptuous, and self-promoting. We feel addicted to

Serve Myself First

VS.

God First, Others Second, & I Am Third

whatever satisfies our selfish desires. With the truth of the gospel, grace is offered to produce change in our lives. Thus, we have the hope of a changed "fruit cycle." We're offered a gracious path of wisdom that produces new fruit in our lives rather than the deadly path of folly that results in addiction. We must pray to the true Savior, Jesus Christ, because we need to be saved from our cycle of sin. Christ and his grace alone can give us insight, strength, and a new heart to break the bondage of our sin cycle. We must cry out for grace because we cannot change our own hearts.

There are two sides to understanding change, which work together as we seek to grow and change our behaviors. The first side is seeing our desperate need for a Savior and for grace to change; the other is our responsibility to make active changes and new choices in our life through steps of faith and obedience.

TWO SIDES OF CHANGE

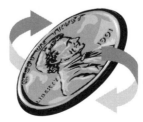

Works - Active Change
Because Christ dwells in me, I have his power to make active changes in my life. I'm responsible for making wise lifestyle choices that glorify and image him the way he intended.

Grace - Passive Change
God changes me through and by his Holy Spirit. I must seek God in prayer, asking that the gift of his Spirit be made manifest in my heart and life. I must ask God to give me eyes to see and ears to hear. I cannot change myself.

The goal of change is that through grace alone, we may fulfill the law of love, which Jesus identified as the greatest of the commandments: "'And you shall love the Lord your God with all your heart and with all your soul and with all your mind and with all your strength.' The second is this: 'Love your neighbor as yourself.' There is no commandment greater than these" (Mark 12:30–31).

SESSION 17
TEMPTATION, FAITHFULNESS, AND CHANGE

KEY CONCEPT: Temptation is a form of suffering we all will face while we live on this earth. God promises to be faithful to rescue us from temptation. He will always provide a way of escape, and yet he also commands us to walk in wisdom by fleeing temptation. God gloriously gives victory and freedom from the pull of temptations as we increasingly turn to Christ and away from the focus of our temptations. God is faithful to bring true change into our lives and enables our growth in faithfulness to him.

SESSION 17—TEMPTATION, FAITHFULNESS, AND CHANGE

Review and Reflect (15 minutes)

Open in prayer. Read last week's Key Concept aloud, and then discuss the questions that follow.

Last Week's Key Concept: Life-dominating sin patterns don't form overnight, and sexual addiction and entrenched patterns of relating are no different. Repeated actions become habits over time. As we've explored in earlier lessons, our actions are the expression of our hearts. Our hearts flow toward enslaving, habitual sin patterns or toward an emerging pattern of life that is increasingly free, holy, and Christlike.

1. How were you helped or encouraged by reading "The Two Sides of Change"?

2. What insights did you gain as you studied the Carnes model? What are you learning about how to respond differently to your triggers?

Exploring the Key Issue (60 minutes)

Read the Key Concept and the section that follows, and then discuss the questions afterward.

Key Concept: Temptation is a form of suffering we all will face while we live on this earth. God promises to be faithful to rescue us from temptation. He will always provide a way of escape, and yet he also commands us to walk in wisdom by fleeing temptation. God gloriously gives victory and freedom from the pull of temptations as we increasingly turn to Christ, and away from the focus of our temptations. God is faithful to bring true change into our lives, and enables our growth in faithfulness to him.

"No temptation has overtaken you that is not common to man. God is faithful, and he will not let you be tempted beyond your ability, but with the temptation he will also provide the way of escape, that you may be able to endure it. Therefore, my beloved, flee from idolatry" (1 Corinthians 10:13–14). Paul wrote these words to encourage the Corinthian believers in their faith and their battles against temptation. He calls temptation "common." And yet so often, Christians sink into shame and discouragement when they encounter lustful thoughts, a craving for a person's attention, or the lure to visit an unholy website. But are these experiences *sin?* The line between temptation and sin can seem blurry. But when we view both from a biblical lens; we see that temptation is not sin, unless *acted upon* with sinful thoughts, behaviors, and desires.

> There are at least three ways that God's goodness can be found even in times of temptation. First, temptation is an opportunity to know God better! The lusts of our hearts are masquerading as God. They lure, and entice, promising joy, comfort, security, etc. Our sin offers us only what God can deliver. Second, temptation builds spiritual muscle. The Christian life is a fight—there is a reason we are exhorted to put on the whole armor of God (Ephesians 6:10–20). Third, God meets us in our temptation and as a result we learn to love Him more.[11]

The glorious promise of 1 Corinthians 10:13–14 is that our faithful God is with us in the battle against temptation and offers us himself as the ultimate way of escape!

3. How do the three aspects of God's goodness in the quote above encourage you in your battle against temptation?

4. Read James 1:15–17. How does the process that James describes relate to Carnes's Cycle of Sexual Addiction, especially in terms of your own sexual or relational sin pattern?

Read the following aloud, and then discuss the questions that follow.

Our battle with particular temptations may be lifelong, but it's one that we're called to engage in through Jesus and alongside other believers. God doesn't promise to take temptation away, but he *does* promise to be there as a comforter, sustainer, and grace-giver. Accepting that we will probably battle certain temptations throughout our lives, whatever they may be, draws us nearer to God and points us to our constant need of a Savior. Jesus saves us not only from the penalty of sin through salvation, but desires to rescue us daily from our own sinful desires and temptations that come against us as we live in this world.

Last week we explored Carnes's Cycle of Sexual Addiction. Now, let's consider another model, which will help us take active steps of wisdom and obedience. Consider how this second model below, and its stages of faith and obedience, compares with the cycle of addictive sin. This model starts from our heart-set of surrender to the Lord, as Lord in our lives. As Lord, he is also the one who dwells within us and gives grace by the power of the Holy Spirit to walk in the ways of God (Galatians 5:16–17, 25).

HOW CHRIST CHANGES OUR PATTERNS OF RESPONSE

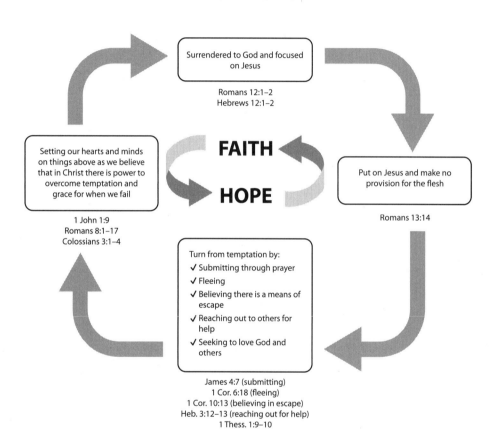

Surrendered to God and focused on Jesus

Romans 12:1–2
Hebrews 12:1–2

Setting our hearts and minds on things above as we believe that in Christ there is power to overcome temptation and grace for when we fail

1 John 1:9
Romans 8:1–17
Colossians 3:1–4

FAITH

HOPE

Put on Jesus and make no provision for the flesh

Romans 13:14

Turn from temptation by:
✔ Submitting through prayer
✔ Fleeing
✔ Believing there is a means of escape
✔ Reaching out to others for help
✔ Seeking to love God and others

James 4:7 (submitting)
1 Cor. 6:18 (fleeing)
1 Cor. 10:13 (believing in escape)
Heb. 3:12–13 (reaching out for help)
1 Thess. 1:9–10

© Ellen Dykas, Harvest USA, 2012

5. What would it mean to be focused on Jesus, rather than being preoccupied with tempting memories, unholy images, etc.?

6. What does it mean to you to "put on Jesus and make no provision for the flesh in regard to its lusts"?

7. Which of the five aspects of turning from temptation (bottom center of model) are the most challenging to you? Why?

Making It Personal (10 minutes)

Read the following silently.

Temptation versus sin . . . it can be a huge turning point to realize the difference between the two. We'll always be tempted by sin(s), present and past, but the vulnerability to that temptation will decrease over time as we learn to repent and take hold of the grace given to us by our Savior. It's important to remember that our temptations and sins don't define us, nor are they our identity. We'll still experience temptation to wrong patterns of relating, certain types of relationships, and other false comforts, but in Christ we are no longer to see ourselves as we once defined ourselves (whore, slut, abnormal, cheap, gay, etc.). In Christ we are sinners, yes, but sinners who have a Savior who identifies us as forgiven and loved daughters of God, and a rescuer who empowers us to battle our besetting temptations.

When we experience a trigger—whether it's loneliness, boredom, anger, tiredness, or emotional pain—we'll experience the temptation to return to the familiar ways of the past with which we soothed ourselves. Our sexual and relational false comforts, and the patterns of thinking associated with them, provided an escape from life for us that was devoid of Christ. The world, our flesh, and the devil will use what worked in the past to tempt us to use it again to ease our trigger, to soothe our discomfort—and later on, numb our discouragement over feeling defeated by the same sin.

Therefore, we must not become devastated or discouraged that we are still tempted; we must persevere in the midst of our temptation. We now have a new choice, a new strength, a way out of our temptations. We don't have to give in any longer. In order to exercise wisdom when seeking a way out of temptation, we must be practical. We must have a behavior plan when temptations do arise. Therefore, we must think ahead of time about what to do when our triggers are tempting us, so that we can begin a new cycle of change instead of reentering our old addictive cycle.

This is a great time to consider a time of intentional abstaining from all sexual expression/activity, and perhaps certain people and social situations as well. A suggested time frame is 90 days. If you've been abstaining from sex, this may also be a good time to think about taking a 90-day break from a specific person (if you're not married) with whom you have an unhealthy or dependent relationship. This means *no contact of any type* for 90 days. This isn't an assignment, but it's something you should seriously consider doing at a point in time *when you're realistically ready to take this step*. Abstaining, or fasting, from triggers that have been connected to sinful patterns can bring clarity and strength to our desire to walk in new paths of obedience and holiness. Consult with your counselor, mentor, and/or spouse before you begin. Seek their advice and their support.

On Your Own (5 minutes)

Complete the following reflective questions and journaling. Come to the next session prepared to discuss your answers.

1. Where do you sense God has strengthened you to "battle well" against temptation? In what areas do you know you're weak and need to be more purposeful in growing?

2. Study the chart from this session, "How Christ Changes Our Patterns of Response." What are specific steps of obedience you can take in view of each aspect of this change process? What can you do to:

- Focus on Jesus?
- Put Jesus on and make no provision for your flesh?
- Flee when temptation is right in front of you?
- Seek others' help when temptation comes, and be honest about your struggles?
- Nurture a mindset on things above, rather than earthly things? How can you sow to the Spirit, watering seeds of godliness in your life?

3. In *Made to Crave: Satisfying Your Deepest Desire with God, Not Food,* author Lysa TerKeurst discusses the process God has taken her through in being freed from sinful eating. Food addiction is similar to people addiction in that we can't just "go cold turkey" off either for life! We need to learn how to enjoy the gift as it is in its proper place in our lives. With people, we need to learn to love and serve; we also need wisdom and discernment to know what

kinds of people, or even specific people, are not safe for us. TerKeurst says, *"My brokenness cannot support [certain types] of freedom. Therefore, I had to flee. I had to remove myself from the source of temptation and I had to do it immediately"* (p. 145, emphasis added).[12]

Are there ways that your brokenness cannot handle certain kinds of relational freedoms right now? Are there individuals, social gatherings, social media connections that you must flee? Journal out your thoughts.

4. Read the testimony below, and journal or list out your thoughts, feelings, and reactions to it. The author is a woman who has battled against the temptation of same-sex attraction. If homosexuality is not a temptation for you, ponder what she says in light of your specific battles of heart, thought, and body.

"Aren't you really still attracted to women?"

The change question: Am I really "changed," or am I still attracted to women? I could write a book about this, but I'll begin by saying that I have not arrived at a place of "no longer tempted" or "no longer able to give way to sin." Personally, I don't think anyone who once indulged in homosexuality and has chosen to leave it will live free of same-sex *temptations*. However, I do believe there is a significant difference between temptation and actually indulging or allowing myself to give into temptation and acting out in a sinful way. I believe temptations are just that—temptations, and nothing more. My temptation does not define me. It is not my identity, nor is it sin. Now, if I acted upon my temptations in ways that are outside God's paths, they're no longer temptations but sin. My temptation has given birth to behaviors that usually quickly envelop my life.

So back to the question: Am I still attracted to women? No and yes. Am I attracted in the sense that I want to have sex with women? No, not anymore. I'm not a light switch; it took time to work through many issues to reach this point. This is where I would distinguish between attraction and admiration. I believe admiration to be the healthy desire or interaction for those of the same sex, and that it is a natural part of friendship. For those of us who struggle with same-sex attraction, this feeling of admiration has for many reasons become romanticized and sexualized. My admiration of women turned into sexual attraction around puberty when the two feelings became mixed together. As an adolescent I would admire a woman, but before I knew it this admiration would become sexualized. I desired closeness, but as an adolescent sexual feeling got thrown into the mix. So emotional intimacy with women became associated with sexualized thoughts and relating.

Fast forward to today . . . Do I admire certain types of women? Yes. Could this admiration turn into attraction? Yes. Do these women have a "theme" about them, or specific traits that draw me to them? Yes. So am I really attracted to that woman or am I attracted to that particular trait, that relational quality she has that I want to get close to or possess in some way? I believe it is the latter.

I believe there were many reasons why I found particular women sexually attractive. It may have felt like I've always been attracted to women, but in reality, I can see that there were reasons beyond sexuality. There have been many contributing influences (soil issues) that helped me to lean toward same-sex attraction—gender detachment, anger issues, fear issues, trauma issues, and issues of feeling separated from the world of women, which taught me all the more to crave and lust for emotional and physical closeness to women. I could go on, but the bottom line is: Attraction is not a simple genital thing. I believe, and can see in my own life, that attraction has many levels and many reasons. For me, coming to understand why I became attracted to certain women has been a key part of the process toward growing and rebuilding a healthy admiration for those of the same sex.

So, can I be attracted to a woman? Yes. *Could and have* I been tempted to want to get close to her sexually? Yes, but I see now that it's not because I need to define and call myself a gay woman, but because of what I crave from her. It could be her beauty, her style, her body, or wanting to rescue or save her. Or it could be traits in her that I see myself as not having and wish I did, to the point of wanting to become sexually close to those traits and possess them myself. In many ways, this attraction is jealousy. I envy this very woman I desire to become close to. I want to touch, possess what she has that I believe I don't have and need. Then there are other levels of wanting to find comfort, closeness, acceptance, a sense of power, of safety, belonging, etc. If I see that this particular type of woman will provide these things, I could find myself tempted to want to become closer to her, to become number one in her life. The quickest way to do that is to have sex with her, to become her all, to come to that place of *feeling* safe, comforted, accepted, known, loved, wanted, etc.

Today I can say that I've learned to discern between attraction and admiration of those women (and even men) I am drawn toward. There is hope; there is a place of freedom from attraction. Freedom looks different for each person. Change is a process. Attraction to admiration is a change over time. Victory is not a point in a lifetime, but rather, something which happens over *the course of* a lifetime.

SESSION 18
A RENEWED MIND: OVERCOMING FANTASY AND UNGODLY THINKING

KEY CONCEPT: Our minds are always active. Therefore, they are always needing transformation and to be captured to Christ. The mind has been called the most powerful sex organ we have because, as we think, so flow our behaviors and patterns of life. Thus, to grow in a holy and healthy pattern of life—including our relationships and sexuality—the battle for the mind is crucial. As we grow in having our thought lives submitted to Jesus, our outward lives also begin to change.

SESSION 18—A RENEWED MIND: OVERCOMING FANTASY AND UNGODLY THINKING

Review and Reflect (15 minutes)

Open in prayer. Read last week's Key Concept aloud, and then discuss the questions that follow.

Last Week's Key Concept: Temptation is a form of suffering we all will face while we live on this earth. God promises to be faithful to rescue us from temptation. He will always provide a way of escape, and yet he also commands us to walk in wisdom by fleeing temptation. God gloriously gives victory and freedom from the pull of temptations as we increasingly turn to Christ and away from the focus of our temptations. God is faithful to bring true change into our lives, and enables our growth in faithfulness to him.

1. What practical steps of faith did you come up with as you studied the chart "How Christ Changes Our Patterns of Response"?

2. What struck you from the testimony in the homework? How do you connect with the woman's thoughts about the ongoing battle against temptation and the hope we have in Christ as we engage in this battle?

3. Did you have any insights in applying this quote to your relational world: "*My brokenness cannot support [certain types] of freedom. Therefore, I had to flee. I had to remove myself from the source of temptation and I had to do it immediately*"?

Exploring the Key Issue (60 minutes)

Read the Key Concept and the following text. Discuss the questions afterward.

Key Concept: Our minds are always active. Therefore, they are always needing transformation and to be captured to Christ. The mind has been called the most powerful sex organ we have because, as we think, so flow our behaviors and patterns of life. Thus, to grow in a holy and healthy pattern of life—including our relationships and sexuality—the battle for the mind is crucial. As we grow in having our thought lives submitted to Jesus, our outward lives also begin to change.

While men generally are stereotyped as being more visually oriented then women, consider the romance-novel industry, for which women are the primary consumers. This billion-dollar business flourishes because it enables a woman to create a fantasy world that she longs to have in her real world. The written word works with disordered desires and an active imagination to produce an active and powerful fantasy.

A fantasy life somehow serves to remake "our" universe in a way that serves our desires, lusts, and agenda. What do you daydream about? What are the recurring stories and themes in your daydreams? Do they seemingly just float into your thoughts randomly, or do you actively pursue them through developing, creating, and then finessing a made-up story or scenario in your mind?

The promise of God's Word is that believers "have the mind of Christ" (1 Corinthians 2:16). This means that our thought lives can be transformed by the loving care of Jesus Christ, giving us the amazing gift to be able to think as he thinks! But it takes *time* + *effort* + *grace* + *faith!*

A transformed thought life is absolutely possible, but the battle to take our thoughts captive to the truth of God's Word doesn't happen overnight. This session will guide you to consider practical suggestions in taking those initial steps that lead to a "recaptured" thought life.

4. Do you engage in fantasy, and if so, what are the themes of the stories you create? What's your role in those fantasies? What role, if any, does God play?

5. When did you begin to engage in fantasy, and why (if you remember)? What are the emotional triggers *now* that lead you to retreat into your fantasy world? If you're not aware of a specific fantasy, do you often feel mentally detached, unengaged, or numb? What patterns of thinking seem lodged or immovable in your mind?

6. Read Philippians 4:4–8. What are the commands in this passage of Scripture? What are the promises? How do your fantasies and/or ungodly patterns of thinking run counter to say what Paul says we're to think upon?

7. How would you describe the difference between unholy fantasy and healthy imagination? Give examples, if you can.

Making It Personal (10 minutes)

Read the following aloud, and then close in prayer.

Fantasies provide a window into our hearts, our perceptions of life, and the ways we want life to work. Our fantasies have themes that reveal our ruling desires (roots) and the interpretations of our lives (shoots) that we carry. The danger comes in believing that fantasies are harmless to us and others. Any time we seek to make life work apart from reality, Christ, and the truth of his Word, we're stepping onto a destructive path. The path to a renewed mind will involve a growing awareness of *what* your fantasies are, *how* and *when* you move into them and *how God's truth speaks* into your fantasy. The promise of God's Word is that your mind *can* be renewed and transformed. The gospel is centered on Jesus Christ, a *real* Savior for our *real* lives.

The hope of the gospel gives new spiritual eyesight for all who will believe. One of the promises Jesus offered in Luke 4:18–19 was to give "recovering of sight to the blind." As unsaved people in the kingdom of darkness, our greatest need was to see and believe in Jesus as Savior and worthy Lord. As believers who continue to struggle against temptation and distorted thinking, we still need the truth of God's Word to give us a new lens of seeing life and ourselves.

On Your Own (5 minutes)

Read "Practical Steps for Recapturing Thoughts" below, and then work through the exercise that follows. Journal about how you've been encouraged and challenged by this reading and questions, and how you're experiencing God's Word in new ways. The process of recapturing our minds to Christ and letting go of fantasy will take time and effort but it's doable, through the power of the Holy Spirit.

Practical Steps for Recapturing Thoughts

Second Corinthians 10:3–5 says, "For though we walk in the flesh, we are not waging war according to the flesh. For the weapons of our warfare are not of the flesh but have divine power to destroy strongholds. We destroy arguments and every lofty opinion raised against the knowledge of God, and take every thought captive to obey Christ."

In the context of this passage, "strongholds" are thought patterns, ways of thinking that are so entrenched in us that they have a *strong hold* upon us. These strongholds of thought form the basis for views and interpretations of life that are based on lies rather than the truth of God's Word. Not only are fantasies fueled by faulty shoots, they also keep false beliefs entrenched within us. Fantasies are the fruit of beliefs we have that God's Word is not able to comfort, encourage, strengthen, or provide for us in the midst of real life—that God's love does not satisfy the deepest place of our souls.

How do we tear down these strongholds? How do we demolish destructive fantasies that have become lodged in our imaginations? The above passage gives us some significant clues:

- We grow in our knowledge of God through his Word.
- We grow in awareness of the thoughts, fantasies, and ways of thinking we've "raised against" God's truth, as revealed in his Word.
- We grow in our ability to actively replace sinful thoughts and fantasies (based upon lies and fueled by self) with godly thinking. This is the process of "taking thoughts captive" to the obedience of Christ. By the power of God within us, over time our thoughts are submitted to Christ's truth. They become conformed to him and how he thinks about any given situation.

Follow the steps below, and before the next session journal or list out how this exercise impacted you. What was encouraging? What was challenging? Be ready to share your reflections and insights at the next session.

1. Pray for God to open his Word to you and to give you understanding.

2. Read all of Romans 12. As we've discovered in earlier sessions, this chapter contains rich teaching about a renewed mind and the kind of life (and relating) it will lead to.

3. Journal about this: How does considering yourself a living sacrifice—one fully belonging to God—help you to have a transformed mind free of selfish fantasy? Think about this, for a start: The offering of yourself fully to God is a spiritual act of worship, while addictive thought patterns are evidence of the worship disorder we are all bent toward—*serving ourselves and making life work our way*! Romans 12:3 speaks to our sinful tendency to think very highly of ourselves—and fantasies that revolve around *us* and *our desires* prove the point.

4. Consider one of your fantasies (or a thought pattern that's filled with fear, insecurity, anger, jealousy, etc.), and journal about this: How does it serve *your* purposes rather than God's? How is your fantasy life a fruit of your conformity to the way the world thinks (Romans 12:2)? How is that thought pattern founded in unbelief rather than in belief that God is who is says he is, and that he can do what he says he can do, and that *you are who he says you are*?

5. The renewal of the mind means being cleansed, shaped, and influenced by God's truth rather than your own "truth." How do you think a renewed mind will help you to discern God's good will concerning relationships, sex, fears, insecurities, desires, or sadness that may be a part of your life?

6. Reread Romans 12:9–21. Which of the verses or topics covered in this passage most connects to your fantasy world and unbelieving patterns of thought? For example, does your fantasy revolve around others loving you (verse 9), serving you (verse 10), around revenge (verses 19–21), and/or around evil sexual expressions (verse 9)?

7. How is God calling you to live in your real world of real people and circumstances this week? How do you need his help? Using the verse you connected to in question 6, write out a private prayer to God of at least three or four sentences. Ask him to cause the truth of his Word to shape your thinking and the ways you respond and relate to people this week.

As you've worked through these questions, you may have thought: *Doesn't all this seem rather simplistic, given that it's taken years, maybe even decades, to develop my fantasy world?* Be assured that strongholds of thought and fantasy *can* be torn down and put into submission to Christ. But it will only happen as you faithfully take small, daily steps like those above to apply God's Word to the life of your mind and imagination,

Over the course of this coming week, continue to follow these steps (and use other portions of Scripture, too) as you pray and ask God to help you engage the battle for your mind. Your first prayer might be to ask God to give you the desire to let go of your fantasy, to will *his* will. He delights to hear his daughters call out to him for help (see Psalm 50:15).

The natural bent of our minds is not toward the ways of God, or toward using our minds to glorify him. Write in your journal and begin praying to the Lord every day to renew your mind. Ask him to make you aware of how you use your mind. Ask others in your life to pray this for you as well. Consider using the following scriptures for meditation and memorization: Isaiah 26:3–4; Romans 8:5–8; Romans 12:1–2; 1 Corinthians 2:16; and Philippians 4:4–8.

SESSION 19
HEALTHY FRIENDSHIPS

KEY CONCEPT: Godly friendships are fueled by a commitment to love God and others, rather than serving self and focusing on what we can get from others. The vibrancy of the Christian life is found in faith being expressed through love, service, and sacrifice, and in living for God's purposes. This stands in stark opposition to a life lived in the pursuit of our own satisfaction, no matter what the risks or costs. Growth in Christlikeness spills over into all areas of life—including friendships.

SESSION 19—HEALTHY FRIENDSHIPS

Review and Reflect (15 minutes)

Open in prayer. Read last week's Key Concept aloud, and then discuss the questions that follow.

Last Week's Key Concept: Our minds are always active. Therefore, they are always needing transformation and to be captured to Christ. The mind has been called the most powerful sex organ we have because, as we think, so flow our behaviors and patterns of life. Thus, to grow in a holy and healthy pattern of life—including our relationships and sexuality—the battle for the mind is crucial. As we grow in having our thought lives submitted to Jesus, our outward lives also begin to change.

1. What did you learn from the exercise of taking practical steps to recapture your thoughts? What successes, no matter how small, did you see as you worked through this?

2. What questions or struggles have you had regarding the process of renewing your mind?

Exploring the Key Issue (60 minutes)

Read the Key Concept, and then discuss the questions that follow.

Key Concept: Godly friendships are fueled by a commitment to love God and others, rather than serving self and focusing on what we can get from others. The vibrancy of the Christian life is found in faith being expressed through love, service, and sacrifice, and in living for God's purposes. This stands in stark opposition to a life lived in the pursuit of our own satisfaction, no matter what the risks or costs. Growth in Christlikeness spills over into all areas of life—including friendships.

3. How would you describe your friendships with women? Have you avoided them, or craved their attention? Are your friendships mostly superficial, or do you tend to have one close friendship that consumes your life? What's contributed to your personal patterns of friendship with women?

4. The term *codependency* refers to unhealthy relationships that exert a destructive and obsessive influence. To the best of your understanding, how does Scripture speak to the concept of codependency, or to the dynamic of seeking security, meaning, value, and life in our relationships?

5. What roles or patterns of relating do you see being played out in codependent relationships, including friendships? When two people are consumed with each other and dependent upon one another, what "idols" do they each seem to feed off of?

6. What roles have you typically played in your unhealthy relationships? Do you seek to rescue people, to be the always-available caregiver? Or are you the one seeking to be taken care of by others? How do these roles serve or soothe you? What are the roots and shoots that drive your patterns of relating in these ways?

7. Turn to Appendix F on page 195, and take a few minutes to look over "The Two Trees of Codependency," which depict examples of self-serving relational styles. Then talk about this: Are your own patterns of friendship represented by either or both of these trees?

8. When Jesus is in his worthy place in our life as Lord and Friend, we are able to enjoy others as good gifts and experience the joy of friendship. Why do

you think it's necessary for Jesus to reign in our hearts as Lord in order to have godly, healthy friendships?

Making It Personal (10 minutes)

Read the following aloud, and then spend time in prayer for each other.

For women with a history of unholy and unhealthy relationships, the idea of growth in godly friendships may be another piece of the Christian life that feels overwhelming. When a woman has a history of detaching and attaching emotionally, driven by the emotional buzz she gets, she'll find it challenging to accept the normal ebb and flow of healthy relationships with women. She may feel frustrated or even hurt that the women she reaches out to don't respond by serving her idols and cravings. A woman may discover that she has so been ruled by selfish desires that she really doesn't know how to initiate—much less build—a healthy, godly friendship. It takes time, effort, and patience.

This is yet another place in our lives where Jesus enters in to bring hope, comfort, and wisdom. Pray for each other to grow in taking the next steps of faith toward being a godly woman who grows into a godly friend.

On Your Own (5 minutes)

1. Read the following passages and then journal or list out what they teach concerning godly relationships, including friendships.
   - Galatians 5:13–26
   - Ephesians 4:25–5:21
   - Colossians 3:1–17

2. Review the trees in Appendix F. Draw or sketch out your own "Friendship Tree," featuring what you see as being the characteristics of a godly friend. What would rule her heart? What worldview would she live out of? What would her desires be? What would be the fruit of her life, in terms of thoughts and behaviors? If you need help working through this, read the passages in question 1 again!

3. Read the "The Look and Feel of Godly Friendships" below. Take time to look up the Bible passages and to journal about the points that most encourage you, as well as those that seem most challenging. Ask God to show you two or three specific steps of faith you can take this week. Ask your group leader for ideas if you need help.

The Look and Feel of Godly Friendships

In a godly friendship, Jesus and God's Word are central. The fruits of this holy centricity will be evident over time and will be seen in increasing ways, such as by worshipping, loving, and obeying God when you're together (see Hebrews 10:24). One way of viewing godly friendship is to consider John 15:1–11 and how the branches are to live alongside each other:[13]

- Branches abide in the vine (Jesus), not in each other.
- Branches live alongside each other, not in isolation from each other!
- Knowing that the vine is the true source of life, a wise and loving branch will encourage the other branches to draw life from the vine, rather than attempting to be a *vine-replacement*!

As women live life alongside each other in godly friendship, abiding in Jesus and his Word, here are some of the fruits that are borne out:

- Over time each friend looks, talks, acts, behaves, thinks, and loves more and more like Jesus (Romans 8:28–29; Ephesians 5:1–2).
- Wholehearted, whole-minded love for God flows out into love for the people in each friend's world—family, church, work, neighborhood (Mark 12:29–31).
- Patience, kindness, and forgiveness reign in the midst of disappointment and failure by others to love you well (Colossians 3:12–14).
- Time spent together brings enjoyment of each other in God's presence. (Psalm 116 contains wonderful truths of how we're to live life before God and people.)
- Love-motivated, truth-speaking, and humble confession of weakness and sin lead each to run to Jesus for his grace, love, and power to change (Ephesians 4:15; James 5:16).
- Communication is full of encouragement, truth spoken in love, wisdom, honesty, and correction—not flattery, gossip, or manipulation (Psalm 19:14; Proverbs 12:18; Ephesians 4:29).
- Each challenges the other to live with heart and mind set on things above and to invest time, resources, affections, and relational energy into the kingdom of God, not on temporary pleasures (Colossians 3:1–3).
- A lack of exclusivity invites others into your circle of two and propels you *out* of your circle of two. Many women have a fierce craving to possess others, yet Jesus enables us to get *out of ourselves* so that we aren't consumed with our desires (2 Corinthians 5:14–15).
- Enjoyment of each other and celebrating life together with laughter is a gift from God that allows a friendship to not be a cycle of drama, but rather honest living in a hard world (Psalm 133; James 1:17).

Ultimately, godly friendships encourage us in our relationship with the ultimate friend, Jesus, and help us to love and serve him!

How can you grow away from your selfish patterns of friendship and toward becoming a godly friend? Faith and obedience never leave us only in a place of saying no to sin, but also enable us to say yes to godliness! Ask God to show you how to say yes to growth in Christlikeness in your friendships, and ask others to pray for and encourage you.

4. During the next session you'll be invited to share some of the highlights of what you've learned over the course of this study, as well as your hopes for next steps of growth. So in preparation for your final session, do a personal "Tree Model Review."

Look over the tree you created on p. 20. Only this time, add the ways you've already experienced change in your life over the course of this study. Philippians 1:6 is a wonderful promise: God *will* complete the work he's started in you! It's been said that growth equals moving in a new direction. As we run the race set before us (Hebrews 12:1–2), with our eyes fixed our eyes on Jesus, we can have the wonderful assurance that he is actively conforming us more and more into Christlike women.

SESSION 20
THE JOURNEY AHEAD: FIXED ON JESUS AS YOU RUN YOUR RACE

KEY CONCEPT: The Christian life is compared to a marathon—it is a race finished by someone who keeps a steady pace toward the finish line. Our journey of growth as women desiring to be like Jesus in our relationships and sexuality is a lot like running a marathon. We must persevere and be aware of temptations to quit or get sidetracked. We will be encouraged as we run alongside others heading toward the same finish line. We will be enabled to endure as we set our hope on Christ, fixing our desires upon him. He is with us in the journey, and he will welcome us home when the race is done!

SESSION 20—THE JOURNEY AHEAD: FIXED ON JESUS AS YOU RUN YOUR RACE

Review and Reflect (15 minutes)

Open in prayer. Read last week's Key Concept, and then discuss the questions that follow.

Last Week's Key Concept: Godly friendships are fueled by a commitment to love God and others, rather than serving self and focusing on what we can get from others. The vibrancy of the Christian life is found in faith being expressed through love, service, and sacrifice, and in living for God's purposes. This stands in stark opposition to a life lived in the pursuit of our own satisfaction, no matter what the risks or costs. Growth in Christlikeness spills over into all areas of life—including friendships.

1. Share about your personal "Friendship Tree" with the group. Explain key points of the tree, and why you feel they're key.

2. What principles for friendship stood out to you as you read the homework Bible passages and "The Look and Feel of Godly Friendship"? How so?

Exploring the Key Issue (60 minutes)

Read the Key Concept aloud, and then discuss the questions that follow.

Key Concept: The Christian life is compared to a marathon—it is a race finished by someone who keeps a steady pace toward the finish line. Our journey of growth as women desiring to be like Jesus in our relationships and sexuality is a lot like running a marathon. We must persevere and be aware of temptations to quit or get sidetracked. We will be encouraged as we run alongside others heading toward the same finish line. We will be enabled to endure as we set our hope on Christ, fixing our desires upon him. He is with us in the journey, and he will welcome us home when the race is done!

3. Read Hebrews 12:1–3 together aloud. What have you learned during this study, about each of the following:

- How important it is to throw off everything that hinders your pursuit of Jesus
- The foolishness of continuing to allow ourselves to be entangled in sin
- What it means to run the race of faith, keeping our eyes fixed on Jesus
- The importance of not growing weary in the process of change, although it may be long and slow at times

4. Share some key highlights from your personal Tree Review. How have you grown already? How do you desire to continue growing into a woman who lives surrendered to Jesus, with your relationships and sexuality?

5. How have your views of Jesus and the Bible changed over the course of this study?

Making It Personal (25 minutes)

Read the section below, and then discuss the questions that follow:

Slow and Steady Wins the Race

Those of us who have lived with addictive patterns of sin know what it's like to be dominated by the craving for instant satisfaction our hearts are pulled toward. We've lived life seeking constant highs or intense moments, saying in our hearts "I want _____ and I want it *now*, the way I want it, and I don't care what God says about it." We've sought relationships in order to get that instant emotional or physical fix. This even spills over into the rest of our lives. Some of us have job-hopped, church-hopped, or moved repeatedly throughout life, seeking something new to avoid the pain or the hard work of actually committing and doing relationship. We've learned to attach and detach from people, jobs, family, and circumstances at the drop of a hat! We've bought into the lie of "if it feels good, do it *now!*" We've been impatient and addicted to our own pleasure and comfort.

The hope of the gospel is: Although we haven't been consistent, faithful, committed people . . . God is faithful to *us!* Earlier in this lesson, we considered Hebrews 12:1–2 and its exhortation to run our race—the life of faith while we live on this earth—with our eyes fixed on Jesus and a persevering spirit. This means we must continue to walk forward step by step, with a steady gait, trusting and praying that "the God of peace himself sanctify you completely, and may your whole spirit and soul and body be kept blameless at the coming of our Lord Jesus Christ. He who calls you is faithful; he will surely do it" (1 Thessalonians 5:23–24).

The key to winning a marathon is not sprinting at the beginning, but running with a pace that is slow and steady throughout the entire 26.2 miles. Our journey through our sexual and relational struggles must be approached with the same mentality. Some of us may struggle with our sexual issues until the day we die, facing temptation continually. Others will find complete freedom. Either way, our mentality ought to be rooted in the promise and hope that God, our faithful Father, will complete his work in us; that Jesus Christ will be ever-present to provide a way of escape; and that the wise Spirit of God will be ever-reminding us of the truth of God, filling us, and enabling us to walk more and more as women who reflect the character of Jesus and the image of God in which we were created.

6. What are a few specific areas of growth you want to target over the next one or two months? For the next year? What hindrances or obstacles do you think might challenge you, as you pursue these areas of growth?

7. Share two or three specific prayer requests with the group—and go to the throne of grace together, as you close out this final session!

On Your Own . . . Your Journey Continues! (5 minutes)

This study has ended, but your journey continues as you walk forward in the Lord. Here's one final passage of Scripture for you to be "sent off" with, as you end this season of study and move on into the next season God has for you:

"May the God of hope fill you with all joy and peace in believing, so that by the power of the Holy Spirit you may abound in hope" (Romans 15:13).

APPENDICES

APPENDIX A
GOD'S DESIGN FOR SEXUALITY

By Ellen Dykas, Harvest USA Women's Ministry staff

Scripture says that God makes and gives to his creation the best pleasures. Psalm 16 says, "At your right hand are pleasures forevermore" (Psalm 16:11). Sex, with all its emotional and physical components of pleasure, comes from the mind of God. It was not something man invented in opposition to God's plan. Scripture declares that God designed us to please him and live a life full of lasting pleasures and joys. This is good news, even as we live all of our earthly days in the midst of a battle against sin.

Even though sin has corrupted all good things, much of the goodness of God's work of creation remains. Furthermore, God's work of redemption extends hope to bring joy from despair. We are called to live within the good and right boundaries of God's design. These boundaries exist for our good and for God's glory. As we grow in understanding God's heart, what his boundaries are, and why they are in place, we grow as women who can enjoy his creation and avoid the entanglements of sexual idolatry and sin.

This article is an overview of the biblical view of godly sexuality. Four key points will be addressed: God as creator of sexuality, godly sexuality for those who are married, godly sexuality for the unmarried, and finally, how we help each other live this out.

1. God as creator of sexuality

Key scriptures: Genesis 1–2; Psalm 24:1–2; Romans 11:36; 1 Corinthians 8:5–6; and Colossians 1:16

The Bible reveals God (Father, Son, and Spirit) as not only the Creator of all things but as a Creator who is very interested in how his creation be experienced. Colossians 1:16 says it clearly, "All things were created through him and for him." And all means *all!* He has designed everything about us—personalities, relationships, gender, sexuality, body—to function and be experienced in a certain way.

Sexuality refers to us as sexual beings who are capable of sexual expression. Our expression can be godly (within God's boundaries) or ungodly (outside God's boundaries and called "sexual sin").

As Creator, God alone has the right to design how his creation is meant to function. The ultimate goal in the design and function of his creation is his glory, a glory that displays the radiance of his holiness, love, goodness, power, etc. We glorify God as we live in a way that reveals who he truly is—worthy of our worship, love, trust, service, and obedience. To put it another way, to give God glory is to acknowledge that he has ultimate weight or significance in our lives, that his word is the anchor by which we live out those lives. God's design for sexuality is a way for him to be glorified by us and through us. 1 Corinthians 10:31 says, "So whether you eat or drink, or whatever you do, do all to the glory of God." Because we exist completely for him and through him, our bodies and sexual lives are also meant to give God glory.

God's glory is also eternally tied to our good. This is important to understand in the context of his design for human sexuality, which God created to be expressed in specific ways. It is not a free-for-all, and yet his wise guardrails are misinterpreted by some as coming from a withholding, prudish, and joy-killing God. This simply is not true. God is good, loving, kind, and cares for us as Father. As our Father who knows our temptations and is merciful toward us as we battle against sinful desires, the boundaries he has put in place for sexual expression are not only for his glory but our protection and flourishing.

2. Godly sexuality for the married   *Doesn't feel fair if you are single.*

Key scriptures: Ephesians 5:22–35; Hebrews 13:4; Song of Solomon

Many people aren't comfortable talking about the beauty, pleasure, and goodness of sex, and God, at the same time! Yet, sex is God's idea . . . his creation in fact! He is glorified and delights in people (the masterpiece of his creation) enjoying good sex, which is godly, Christ-honoring sexual expression. God's blessed context for sexual expression is marriage. Marriage, as created and designed by God, is a lifelong, committed union between one man and one woman.

Godly sexuality within marriage is a way for God to be glorified and for a husband and wife to experience the joys and pleasures of God's creation.

Sexual activity within marriage, experienced as God has designed, reveals and points to him as the giver of good gifts for the delight of his children.

Sex within marriage is:

a. For God-blessed pleasure and delight, but never our selfish desires or demands.

b. An opportunity to honor and love someone above yourself.

c. An opportunity to participate in creating.

d. A bonding experience that echoes the union of Christ with his people.

e. One of the ways a husband and wife express devotion to Christ, through commitment to their marriage covenant, which calls them to complete faithfulness (mentally, emotionally, sexually) to one— their spouse.

"Becoming one flesh" within marriage is more satisfying than anything the world offers as a sexually attractive substitute. Like a fire inside a fireplace, it provides light and warmth, but outside the right context sex can destroy, like an un-extinguished cigarette can burn down a huge forest. Sex is not the purpose of marriage or a good enough reason to get married. Sex is not the goal. It is a means to an end. The Lord gave sexual intimacy, as a natural part of married life, to be an intense, joy-giving way to celebrate and reaffirm covenant love. Rest assured God is very pleased when godly couples enjoy it."[14]

3. Godly sexuality for the unmarried

Key scriptures: Hebrews 13:4; 1 Thessalonians 4:1–8; 1 Corinthians 7:35

Christ offers treasures to all who seek to live in a way that is pleasing to God as image-bearers who are sexual beings, including the unmarried. Godly unmarried sexuality is more than a call to abstain from sexual activity—it is God's context for revealing his glory to and through an unmarried person. While the married person is called to faithfulness to Christ through sexual faithfulness to a spouse, the unmarried person is called to faithfulness to Christ through abstaining from sexual expression. As much as people have tried to "make it work," we just don't see God delighting in and smiling about any type of sex outside marriage (with someone you love but are not married to, sex with self, homosexual, with strangers, with objects or animals).

Godly unmarried sexuality is:

- The reality of being single, but still a sexual being.
- A call to abstinence from sexual expression/activity.
- A way to live out faithfulness and devotion to Jesus, as the unmarried state allows for a unique attending upon Christ.
- An opportunity to honor marriage and keep a future (or potential) marriage bed pure.
- A signpost to Jesus that reveals him as sufficient and worthy of obedience, as expressed by staying within God's boundaries.
- A powerful way to learn how to love people rather than using them for sexual selfishness.
- A wonderful way to prepare for godly *married* sexuality!

4. How we help each other live godly sexual lives

Key scriptures: 1 John 1:7–9; Hebrews 3:12–13; Ephesians 4:15, 29; Hebrews 4:14–16

Living a godly sexual life, whether married or single, is more than difficult—it's impossible without God's grace and empowering presence in our lives! God gives us each other to help one another live out godly sexuality. In this sense, it's a "community commitment."

How can we help each other?

a. We pray for and encourage each other with God's love and truth.

b. We remind each other of the supremacy of Christ over temporary sexual, mental, and emotional pleasures that tempt us to think and act outside God's design.

c. We remind each other that temptation is common, that struggling is normal, and that Jesus rescues and comforts us in our trials.

d. We foster an atmosphere of openness and confession of sin in our relationships. We help each other go to the throne of grace to receive mercy and help because we all need Jesus on a daily basis!

e. We commit to get involved in knowing each other, being known, and asking the hard questions of accountability that spur us to put on the Lord Jesus Christ and make no provision for our flesh.

God's design for sexuality is good and is *for* our good. In order to live out a godly sexuality, we are dependent upon God. Consider, in closing, what our savior and redeemer Jesus Christ offers us as we seek to live within his design. Jesus:

- Gives us himself (John 14:18).
- Names us: *mine, loved, forgiven, a new creation in Christ* (2 Corinthians 5:17).
- Knows and loves us in our temptation (Matthew 26:34–35).
- Enables and empowers us to resist temptation (1 Corinthians 10:13).
- Forgives and restores us when we sinfully give in to temptation (1 John 1:9).
- Gives wisdom and discernment (Colossians 2:3).
- Gives brothers and sisters to help and shepherd us. These brothers and sisters are the body of Christ on earth that he gives to teach, counsel, comfort, guide, and love us (Hebrews 3:12–13; 10:24–25).
- Gives us good works to do that will bear much fruit for his glory. This has everything to do with living as godly sexual beings! We abstain from certain things, but also fully participate in others— including his holy work in this world (Ephesians 2:10; 1 Peter 2:9–10; John 15:5).

APPENDIX B
BROKEN SEXUALITY: WHAT HAPPENS WHEN WE TURN AWAY FROM GOD'S GOOD DESIGN

By Ellen Dykas

What makes sexual sin, *sin*? And what does it mean to call our sexuality "broken"? Our first article, "God's Design for Sexuality" (Appendix A), explains that God the Creator designed our sexuality to be experienced and expressed in certain ways. All people are sexual beings, and thus both the married and unmarried have a form of sexuality. However, in God's good design, all sexual *expression* is meant to be contained within marriage. Marriage, in God's created design, consists of one man with one woman, joined together in a lifelong covenantal union. The good gift of marriage is the context for sexual expression, love for God and neighbor, and lifelong faithfulness to one's spouse. The good gift of singleness is the context for both Christ-enabled abstinence from sexual expression and love for God and neighbor.

Thus, when we live outside God's design for sexuality, we're expressing broken sexuality. Sexuality has become a way we express the idols in our hearts, thus re-creating sex in our own image and calling it "good." Our own disordered desires and definitions of "good" bear themselves out in broken ways. Sex (meaning *all* sexual relating, not only genital-to-genital intercourse) with someone who isn't your spouse, having sex with yourself, or indulging in selfish sexual fantasy, are all ways that sinful hearts express themselves in sexually broken ways. Broken sexuality is:

1) Universal—because sin is universal! Broken sexuality began in Genesis 3, with the fall of man and the introduction of sin into the human race. Sin has impacted every part of our being. It has impacted our bodies, minds, emotions, and desires, as well as our ability to think, reason, and understand. It's important that we acknowledge this because now, due to sin, our impulses and feelings seem very natural, while God's design feels very *un*natural and hard.

Think about it: Is it easier to take the lingering look at a person or image you're sexually aroused by, or to turn away? Is it easier to feel an unholy desire and water it, or to starve it out? Sin feels very natural and easy to us, but that doesn't mean it's holy, right, or "just who we are."

In one sense, sin *is* who we are because of our sin nature. However, in Christ Jesus, we learn how to put the sinful nature to death and to walk out *new* life—Christ in us, the hope of glory (Galatians 5:13–26; Colossians 1:27)! Living out godly sexuality is a lifelong battle for every person, but through the promises of the gospel we have everything we need to live a godly life and escape from sinful sexual desires (2 Peter 1:3–4).

2) Self-centered. Counter to God's call to love and selfless service for his glory, sexual sin demands and pursues several things:

- *I must be at the center of the universe.* My pleasure, comfort, satisfaction, and preferences are what matter most.
- *Now is what's most important.* I can't wait. I shouldn't *have* to wait. And you shouldn't stand in my way. This is one of the effective ways that Internet pornography has nourished self-centered sexuality; it promises and delivers immediate mental sexual pleasure without asking you to lay down your life or to honor anyone above yourself.
- *Escape* from the pain, disappointments, fears, and even boredom we feel as we live in a broken world. We live in an exceedingly pain-intolerant culture. Feeling good and being comfortable are powerful idols that rule many of us. Sexual sin, of any type, is a way that women and men medicate (or numb) their hurting hearts.
- *Avoidance of God, and of true love for others.* Sexual sin detaches us from the love of God and others. Think of the impact of relationships built on sexting, sexual chatting, and random hook-ups. Consider the impact of a monogamous couple who resist the Spirit and give way to their sexual desires for each other outside marriage. And what about the impact of viewing pornography and masturbating? Each of these fuels love for (and slavery to) self, rather than love for God and others by serving, honoring, caring, and walking in obedience.

Broken sexuality is universal, self-centered, and sinful. It is also redeemable, changeable, and forgivable! God's grace, love, cleansing, and forgiveness goes deeper and wider than our sin—including sexual sin. Jesus frees us from ourselves, so that we may truly become what God has created us to be—loved, unashamed, radiant, and godly sexual beings!

APPENDIX C
THOUGHTS ON PARENT-CHILD
BONDING

By Harvest USA Staff

In the fields of psychology and child development, *Attachment Theory* addresses the dynamic of healthy (or unhealthy) bonding between primary caregivers (mainly parents) and children. The theory explains that through our parents we either experience a sense of safety and security ("home") or we don't. When we don't experience safety and security in our home, it often fuels real or perceived experiences of abandonment and rejection. According to this theory, whatever our attachment pattern with our caregivers or parent(s) is, we tend to repeat it later in life in future relationships, or to pursue attaching to (or detaching from) people in unhealthy ways as a means to get what we desired but didn't experience in our formative years. Scripture explains what is at the core of unhealthy attachment patterns we may have: the sinful and broken human heart is always craving and worshipping *something*!

We must realize that even the godliest of mothers will not parent their daughters perfectly, nor will any daughter experience a perfect environment to develop into womanhood. This is the reality of living in a fallen world with fallen people, including parents! It's important to keep in mind that our own hearts are spiritually blind and deceptive (Jeremiah 17:9). These truths do not minimize the deep pain many women feel when honestly assessing their relationship with their moms. It actually leads us to ponder the truest, nurturing love that is available through Jesus Christ, God and Savior.

Fathers generally serve as the first man in a girl's life who influences a rejection or acceptance of her femaleness. He plays a vital role in the development (or absence of development) of a girl being comfortable in being a girl/woman, and also in the development of a woman's view of men being safe and desirable, or not. Dads (and brothers) model the "otherness" of the male gender, and daughters/sisters will experience maleness as different (not superior or inferior) from themselves as female. Just like the most well-intentioned and godly mother, a godly father will not do any of this perfectly. Human families are important *and* imperfect. Thankfully, it's not our family of origin that has the last word—*or the defining word*—about who we are and what we can become!

God's gracious love intervenes, always, for those who will seek to view their lives through the lens of Christ, regardless of their family of origin. As we gain insight into how broken patterns of relating grew out of broken modeling in our childhood, we begin to see the wisdom and truth of God in a fresh light. And conversely, as we grow in our understanding of being *in* Christ Jesus, we better understand our identity as daughters of God. These wonderful truths don't erase the pain we may have experienced due to having imperfect parents, but they do remind us that we need transformed minds and biblical understanding regarding our upbringing (Romans 12:2). God brings wholeness and forgiveness to us, so that we can extend love and forgiveness to others. Our relationship with him is to be our lens through which we view, interpret, and respond to all others.

Changing our patterns of relating to people, including how we attach and bond in healthy, holy ways is a lot like rewiring a house—it's possible, but it's also difficult and messy. When a house is first built, the walls and beams are exposed, making it easy to lay down the electrical wiring. However, once the house is built, pulling out the old wiring and putting in new wire requires making holes in the walls and lots of other internal changes. Yet, as we receive Jesus' promises for us, this is what we must do. We have old wiring—patterns we've learned over time through many influences—that is second nature to us. Through faith and obedience, learning to "put on" Jesus and his ways of relating, and learning to "put off" our sinful nature, we will grow into right ways of doing relationships. This will take time and practice, with new ways of relating to both men and women. Growth in Christlikeness happens over time, but God's Word promises that *we can change* (see Romans 8:28–30).

APPENDIX D
FACING ANGER AND EMOTIONAL PAIN[15]

By Sarah Lipp, former Harvest USA Women's Ministry Staff

A consistent theme for women who battle habitual sexual sins is a parallel struggle of not knowing how to confront and respond to painful circumstances and emotions, such as anger, in a healthy way. Real growth in our lives and relationships happens as we gain awareness of our interior world and pursue change through Jesus Christ. As we wade through the muck and mire of this process and walk in the light with each other, we encourage and help each other to grow.

Anger is an emotion that infects many areas of my own life. The scenarios I'm about to share are obviously from my perspective as a woman; however, I repeatedly hear these same kinds of stories from the women I've counseled, whether they struggle with same-sex or heterosexually-oriented sin, or both. We all act out of our anger and other painful emotions in sinful ways. I hope you'll be able to see yourself in these situations, and I challenge you to wrestle with this whether your struggle with reacting to anger is by binge eating, restricting your eating, isolating, yelling, gossip, biting remarks, etc.

Temptation Rears Its Ugly Head

The first scenario begins with the movie *North Country*, which was based on actual events in Minnesota. Charlize Theron plays a woman named Josey Aimes, who takes a job at the local coal-mining company after divorcing her physically and verbally abusive husband. She takes the job in order to put food on the table and a roof over her children's heads. She and the handful of other women there are repeatedly abused physically, verbally, emotionally, and sexually while working in this predominantly male environment, all the while being told to "take it like a man." One scene showed one of the ladies using a port-a-potty, which was turned over while she was in it. The degradation the women endured by these men was overwhelming, sickening, and obscene. The actual events ended up in a landmark sexual harassment lawsuit, which these ladies won.

I share this with you because during, immediately following, and for days after watching this movie, I began my all-too-familiar cycle of rage—shaking my fist at God, men, and women who excuse the behavior of men as "boys will be boys." A vow from my past crept in my heart: I didn't want to be part of this reality any longer. I said to myself and others, "No wonder I was gay!" I began to rehearse in my heart why I should just go back to women, as old familiar thoughts raced through my mind. Men, and God's design for them, only serve to hurt, use, and abuse women. I reasoned that I was much better off with women, with whom I had experienced safety, value, protection, and significance. This rationalizing allowed my mind to recall old memories, leading me down a road that made me vulnerable to the temptation of my former life. All this took place over a period of three days.

My second scenario revolves around a friendship and a hurtful encounter. I found out that this person had gossiped about things I had shared in confidence with her. Upon finding this out, I felt betrayed, rejected, and abandoned. On the heels of these emotions, I felt a surge of anger. I felt in my heart and resolved in my mind to be done with this person and with those who participated in the gossip. I became furious and felt justified in freezing this person out of my inner circle of friends. I decided this person was dead to me from this point on. Some days after deciding this and fuming about it to friends, I found my mind wandering back to memories of past sexual experiences. I began to feel the loss of being able to live freely as a lesbian when I wanted to. I began to rehearse the reasons of why it's so unfair that I'm restricted by this God I say I believe in, who tells me who I can love and with whom I can be sexually intimate. I became very sensitive to noticing women and men I was sexually drawn to and sensitive to anything that reminded me of the restrictions my faith put upon me.

Anger Is Power

I share these scenarios to unpack how anger is intimately tied to sexual sin. Sexual brokenness, in any form, has a reputation for repeating itself. In fact, anger is frequently listed as a trigger in common addiction models, for both acting out and relapsing. Most of us don't know how to deal with anger, nor how to remain aware of the triggers that lead to an anger that's acted upon through sexual sin (whether the acting out is done shortly thereafter or years later). I believe it's crucial for us to understand the link between our anger and our sexual sin.

Scripture describes a link between anger and sin. Specifically, James 4:1–3 speaks of conflicts resulting from our desires that are thwarted in some way. Then, out of our hearts, anger gives birth to sinful lusts and longings that bring about more conflict. The anger feels powerful, and while it soothes our pain, it results in self-serving and destructive behavior (Matthew 15:18–20).

Anger is a two-sided coin. One side is the raw feeling of anger; the other side is the painful feeling of hurt and disappointment. These two sides, working together, are often an overlooked aspect of the path that leads toward sexual sin. To feel emotional pain when your desires have been dashed is normal and human! Experiences of rejection, abandonment, and betrayal—or of being used, unseen, unknown, uncared for, insignificant, and not safe (emotionally and/or physically)—are painful, and they do sting! I felt all these emotions as I watched and reflected upon the movie and my own painful experience with my friend.

It's important to note that feeling hurt can lead either to holy anger or sinful anger. Throughout my life I was both angry and hurt by the reality that men would treat women so sadistically, and use and abuse them with no conscience. I was hurt that my God allowed such atrocities to occur. I was hurt by the women that turned a blind eye and excused it all. I was hurt by feeling betrayed and abandoned by those who I thought were my friends. I was hurt, and that hurt turned into anger. And yet pain, disappointment, and anger are in some sense legitimate responses to a broken and fallen world, where people use and are used by one another. In this world I wanted to experience trust, respect, love, kindness, and protection from others, but those hopes and desires were thwarted. Anger and pain was the currency I used to act out sinfully.

How does this happen? How does right anger and legitimate hurt turn into an active pursuit of homosexual or heterosexual sex, or lead to relationships that end in destruction? Those of us who have misused sex—whether it has become an addiction or not—must acknowledge that we've had a pattern of using sex to soothe emotions that lead us to feel out of control, powerless, lonely, uncomfortable, and angry. I have used sex in my mind, my desires, and ultimately my actions to create a world where I felt wanted, loved, seen, powerful, safe, and secure—a warm and fuzzy world I could escape to and numb feelings I didn't want to feel. I've always felt safe and powerful to admit my anger. However, anger is like a lead dog on a dogsled; it is connected to other strong emotions that both pull and drive my heart. Anger drove that emotional sled so that I could escape from feeling hurt, wounded, or weak. Sexually acting out was the destination my anger led to—a place where I could escape the pain and once again feel safe, loved, and powerful.

Sucking the Thumb of Sinful Anger

A former colleague of mine had a statue of Linus from the Charlie Brown cartoon in his office. If you'll recall, Linus is the little boy who carries his baby blanket around and sucks his thumb all the time. The image of Linus, with his blanket and thumb-sucking habit, is a visual reminder of what sexual sin is all about. It is about responding in childish ways to life in a fallen world. I can be just like Linus. When life gets hard—when I feel things that make me uncomfortable, when I face conflict, when I can't get my own way or live like I want—I run to my baby blanket, sucking my familiar thumbs of sex, overeating, under eating, isolation, criticalness, gossip, anger, masturbation, overworking, laziness, passivity, etc. I then react to my world in childish ways and with child-level coping skills—numbing, avoiding, and seeking self-gratification—rather than in mature and wise ways.

The progression of sinful anger may take seconds, minutes, days, or months to lead someone to pursue sexually sinful behaviors. It may look something like this:

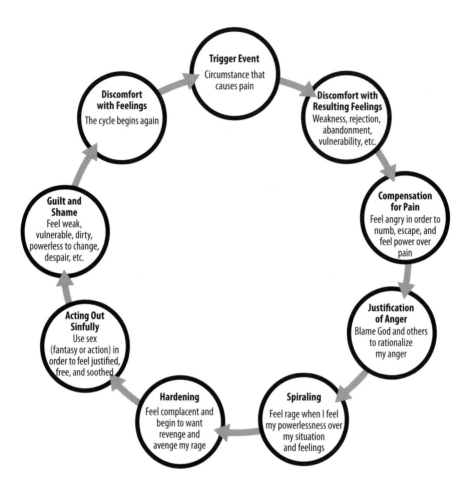

So what are mature and wise ways of coping in a fallen world and dealing with feeling hurt, vulnerable, weak, and raw? I propose that it's to feel (not avoid) the whole spectrum of our emotions, grow in our ability to communicate on a heart level, and flee lust through loving others.

Facing My Emotions

So how do we do this? First, we need to base our emotions and behavior on the scriptural premise that God calls us to live in light and in truth (1 John 1). God calls us to live in the land of reality, rather than pursue whatever it takes to numb our anger and other painful emotions. In God's design, it's appropriate to feel what we feel. We're human, and our emotions were hardwired into us so that we might interpret what we experience in this world. Our interpretation of these emotions have become flawed by the fall; nevertheless God, through his restorative redemptive work through Jesus, gives us grace to grow in navigating our emotions. Through Jesus, we can more fully feel our emotions, more clearly interpret them, and allow them to teach us to respond in godly ways.

Those of us who have used sex as a soothing life response to strong emotions tend to stuff emotions internally. We learned early on that sex was the one way we could safely feel our emotions. We bought into the lie that it shows weakness to reveal to others or to ourselves that we feel hurt, lonely, rejected, abandoned, or like a failure—and weakness is to be avoided at all costs. So we faced life with this enduring thought: Never appear or admit you're weak. It's too dangerous. Sex became an island of escape where we could finally feel deeply, feel free to feel, and feel free to receive feelings from someone else.

How many of us have said or felt before acting out sexually: "I just need to relax"; "I want to feel loved"; "I want to feel wanted, accepted, important to someone"; "I don't want to feel this loneliness"; "I want to feel seen," etc.?

Acknowledging and letting myself feel my emotions needs to be rooted in my ability to trust and rest in Jesus. Believing that he is my God who not only created my emotions but experienced them in the flesh (just like me) gives me hope that I won't be destroyed by them. He does not see me as weak when I cry out (Hebrews 4). Jesus allowed himself to feel emotion. Jesus felt loss, abandonment, pain, and betrayal (Luke 19:41; John 11:35; Matthew 9:36, 26:37–38; Mark 14:42). To face and constructively deal with my emotions is to follow the example of Christ. Feeling my emotions and not becoming ruled by them is imaging and imitating God himself. Practically, this means acknowledging what I'm feeling and taking the time to dig deeper into understanding *why* I'm feeling these emotions. As I do so, I break down walls that have kept me in control and allow myself to feel and unpack my pain, instead of trying to escape, numb, or avoid it. This leads me to the second outlet of facing my emotions:

Communication

Communicating our innermost feelings—the ones we avoid—lies in the gospel call to confess our sins to one another. By truthfully expressing who we are and what we're going through, we allow the community around us to help carry our burdens (James 5:13–20; Galatians 6:2). Here I expose my weak and vulnerable heart to Jesus and others.

Communicating on a heart level is about taking those feelings I now allow myself to feel and articulating them *out loud*! This means that when I feel angry, lonely, hurt, or frustrated, I actually open my mouth and communicate that to the person I'm feeling it toward—and with Jesus too. I must learn how to communicate with those in my everyday life here on earth, and with my Confidant in heaven, about everyday matters as well as matters of the heart.

Those of us who have lived life stuffing our emotions are people who have avoided conflict *at all costs*. When we've felt conflict or hurt, we've detached and moved on rather than confronted the person and shared our feelings about the situation. We avoided or ran from doing the hard work of relationship. We avoided the possibility of working through uncomfortable feelings we have toward people and situations. We avoided praying for discernment and courage to reach out and heal relationships honestly.

Having a sexual and/or emotionally enmeshed relationship is easy because it revolves around seeking to satisfy the needs of another person and to be filled up by that person, for my benefit. However, these kinds of relationships suck the life out of each person rather than give life. They're all about feeling safe and comforted—that warm fuzzy "living on an island" feeling at all times. Holy and healthy relating means that we seek to grow in loving others, both in and through the hard and uncomfortable situations that arise, rather than using them to be filled up or feel safe. As we allow the life of Christ within us to empower us and receive the satisfaction that he alone gives, we have the grace we need to work through conflict and not run to the Band-Aid of codependency or sex.

True relational communication is grounded in my trust that God is who he says he is—a good God who hears, listens, and is able to handle my emotional words. Jesus is my confidant, my husband, my best friend— all roles that require honest and revealing communication. This foundation brings communication that fosters life, freedom, respect, and encouragement to others. Because the Lord chose to open my deaf ears and communicate life to me, I choose to work through my feelings of hurt, discomfort, and conflict by communicating verbally rather than sexually, and by pursuing redemptive, healthy relationships with others. The result is true relationship, rather than unhealthy emotional dependency or sinful sexual relating.

Loving Others

The third component of wise and mature relating is committing to love others as an expression of love for God. Many of us who have sought out sex and enmeshed relationships as a way to control the uncertainty and pain of life have few true, healthy friendships, if any. We have lived by intimately connecting to only one person at a time—the person we're having sexual contact and/or complete emotional enmeshing with. Because the unhealthy fusion to another person takes all our time, energy, and resources, it becomes nearly impossible to significantly connect and communicate with anyone else. We isolate our lives to one person at a time, and when that relationship has ended we're completely isolated and alone again. We haven't understood how to have friends at a heart level without instantly guaranteeing the safety of that relationship (or so we believe) through sex. This is what the Bible calls idolatry. We have worshipped relationships and what that other person is able to provide us. This intense worship, not of God but of other people, is rooted in self-centeredness. Typically, therefore, it causes us to forsake the community of the church—the very place in which, by worshiping the true God, we grow and learn how to authentically and selflessly love others (Hebrews 10:24–25).

Ultimately, the way out of this destructive relationship cycle is to reengage our love for God (the vertical plane) and others (the horizontal plane). Jesus taught that there are two commandments that summarize God's plan for his people—to love God and to love others as I love myself (Matthew 22:37–40). Loving others is always the solution to destructive lust and unhealthy relationships. Loving another from a Christlike, biblical perspective means unclenching our fists, stopping our cries of "It's unfair!" and committing to love and serve others. Because of the passionate love Jesus has for me, and I for him, I'm able to take the energy I poured into justifying my anger, lust, and pursuit of sexual sin and use it to serve others first rather than myself.

At this point, I often hear the cry, "But I can't love others because obviously I can't love myself!" The fact is: Even if it's destructive, you *are* loving yourself. You're pouring your entire life into making yourself feel better *at all costs*! We love ourselves all the time—and that doesn't mean we pamper ourselves in a nice hotel! It means my whole life focus—my energy, my resources, my time—is all spent on *me*, no matter if it hurts me or anyone else! Imagine the incredible change that would happen if you focused your energy on loving and blessing others in life-giving ways, rather than soothing yourself!

We have been living incredibly selfish, self-sufficient, self-focused, self-reliant, and ultimately *destructive* lives. We rarely, if ever, focus on serving or loving anyone else. It may look like we're serving or loving others, but really we're making life more comfortable for ourselves by avoiding conflict (or whatever) so we can have peace; manipulating others for praise or acceptance; serving someone so we feel a sense of power; or serving so we can receive security in return. We spend our lives soothing ourselves through the most convenient and familiar ways we know how. We've been doing what works and what is most comfortable for us because it's too risky to love someone else. Loving someone else means putting my time, energy, desires, resources, and reputation on the line—putting Jesus first, others second, and me last. It's laying down my rights, my anger, my hurt, my comfort, my safety, my pleasure, my significance, and my vengeance. I am not God, I am not king, I have no rights, if I have become a servant of Jesus Christ.

God's invitation to come to his throne of grace (Hebrews 4:16) when I'm hurting, needy, or angry is the draw that leads me to turn from self and using others, and instead seek to love others. Really believing and worshipping Jesus as the Son of a *good* God—who takes the anger and vengeance I deserve and turns it into eternal acceptance, love, and forgiveness—changes my heart to want to worship and follow him in my sexuality, emotions, thoughts, communication . . . my whole life. The grace Jesus Christ gives me disarms my sinful anger and leaves the tank of my destructive lust empty.

APPENDIX E
COMMON LIES

Common Lies about God and My Sin

By Harvest USA Staff

The lies and messages we believe are like breathing—we don't even think about them. They've become automatic tapes playing over and over in our thoughts. Therefore, it's hard to become cognizant of them and then to learn to replace them with the truths of God's Word. This process takes time and diligence, but it's possible!

We are interpreters of our world. We behave the way we do because we've developed an interpretation of the world based on what's happened to us and how we've responded. We've developed beliefs about God, parents, church, friends, relationships, gender, sex, society, men and women, etc., to help us get through life. In order to break our destructive and unholy patterns of relating to others, we must name the lies and replace the false messages and interpretations that we believe. As we grow in faith and knowledge of God's ways, our worldview becomes more and more aligned with God's view for all areas of our lives. Here are just some of the common lies women may believe, as well as God's truth that we can begin learning to apply.

God is out to punish and shame me whenever I sin . . . especially **this sin.**

The Lie: We believe God is an angry God, due to legalistic thinking or perhaps messages we received growing up. We buy into the lie that we must do certain things to be living right. We believe we dare not sin—and if we do, there is a hierarchy of sin with certain types receiving more wrath from God than others. Sexual sins—whether homosexual, heterosexual, or solo—will result in God punishing us and perhaps rejecting us.

The Truth: When we believe this lie, we proclaim God to be unmerciful, rather than abounding in grace or forgiveness. This lie keeps us in a life of penance or a mindset of reward and punishment, driven by fear of a caricature of God rather than the true God. If we commit a sexual sin, we believe we must receive punishment to atone or balance out our sin. The truth is, Christ's sacrifice is sufficient for any and all sins we commit (2 Corinthians 12:9; Hebrews 10:10; 1 Peter 3:18). The Bible is clear that God accepts, loves, and forgives sexual sinners (Luke 7:36–50; John 4:1–30; 8:1–11). God considers all sin equally and lists sexual sins on the same level as other sins such as gossip, stealing, and anger (1 Corinthians 6:9–11; Galatians 5:19–21). He is a God of love who desires to forgive (Matthew 18:12–14; John 3:16). God's punishment only comes on those who refuse to turn to their loving Lord for forgiveness of sin.

God thinks sinful sexual behavior is the ugliest of all; therefore, he sees me as ugly and unforgiveable.

The Lie: If our struggle has been with homosexual desires and acts, we may have been told that this is a sure ticket to hell. We've identified ourselves by our sin: "I sin in a homosexual way, therefore I am homosexual." Or, "I identify on the inside with the male gender, therefore I am gay." "Since I'm gay and homosexuality is the sin of all sins, God must hate me." If our struggle has been heterosexual in nature, we've heard words like "whore" and "slut." We believe that even if God's love is real, it's not strong or deep enough to extend to a sexually broken woman.

The Truth: We are not our sin; our sin does not define us. Believers are forgiven and given a new name, no matter what their besetting sins are (2 Corinthians 5:17; 1 Peter 2:9–10). We may struggle with our sexuality, but our sin or sexual struggle is *not our name or identity*. People do not go to hell for struggling with sexual sin, but for refusing to believe in Jesus Christ and worship him as God (John 14:6; Romans 1:21–25; 1 Corinthians 6:11; Ephesians 2:4–10).

God is unfair, not good, distant, and cruel.

The Lie: We believe that God doesn't really care about us. He may have made everything, but he is not interested in it, nor in us and what we experience. He delights in taking away things we love and cherish. On top of all this, God seems very much like the "big *man* in the sky" who has made life miserable for women. Why trust such a God?

The Truth: We may feel this way for a number of reasons: Life seems cruel, especially if we've experienced any form of sexual abuse or have a struggle with same-sex attraction. We think that if God didn't have these rules against certain sexual behaviors, we could be happy, have who we want, and do what we want. Yet these beliefs come out of a confused understanding of God and the impact of sin on the universe. Human sin has caused the pain and suffering we experience. Evil and injustice in the world are the result of sin, not ignorance or misunderstanding alone. God is perfect and holy and *must* punish sin. To overlook sin would imply that it doesn't matter what we do, and that God is not interested in eradicating evil and injustice. But God is just and holy as well as merciful. He cares so much about restoring what was broken by sin that he sacrificed his own Son, Jesus Christ, to make the payment for our sins (Romans 5:8). Instead of condemning the whole world for its evil, he shows his love by sacrificing a substitute, Jesus Christ, so that we might be forgiven (Romans 3:23–26) and enjoy relationship with him. While we still live in a sinful world, where we both sin and are sinned against, God has provided an amazing solution for our sin problem, at great cost. He shows his righteous judgment against sin by requiring payment, and reveals his gracious love through the death of Jesus, which secures salvation for all who believe in him (John 3:16; 1 John 4:10).

God is just like my dad.

The Lie: The concept of a Father God is repugnant! Fathers are authoritarian, unjust, and abusive. Fathers are distant, cold, and couldn't care less about us. Why would I want to believe in a God like *that*?

The Truth: Our view of God as a father is distorted by how we view our human fathers. However, God *is not* our earthly father. God is neither male nor female, as men and women are, but the Creator of them both. Genesis 1:27 states that both male and female are the image of God. In John 4:24, Jesus states that God is a spirit and must be worshipped in spirit and truth. Our understanding of God may become distorted because of our experiences with our own father or with men in general, but we must not "re-image" God in any way we want, just because it might suit our own needs.

While it is hard to escape the experiences, hurts, and disappointments we may have had with our fathers, it is important not to project these things onto God. The Father revealed in the Bible is one who forgives, pursues, accepts, and loves his children (Psalm 130:3–4; Luke 15:20; 1 John 4:8b–11). Instead of rejecting God because of our imperfect and sinful earthly fathers, we should reject the lies we've embraced based upon our relationships with them.

God helps those who help themselves.

The Lie: God has high expectations of people, and we must work hard to meet them. The person who does not strive to better herself will ultimately fail and be displeasing to God. God only helps us when we work to help ourselves. Being saved, accepted, and forgiven is dependent upon us. We must do right, *or else*. Our standing with God is dependent upon religious works and our best efforts to be a good person.

The Truth: This is the lie of legalism—that we can be good enough in ourselves, by constant self-improvement, to earn God's favor. This is a denial of the gospel and rejects the scriptural perspective that it is God who saves us and grows us, by his grace alone, through faith in Christ alone (Ephesians 2:4–10). The gospel is a message of extravagant grace and love: God lovingly does for us what we cannot do for ourselves. By sending Jesus to die in our place, God gives us his power to grow and change to live according to his design. We cannot change ourselves to earn his favor. "[B]ut God shows his own love for us in that while we were still sinners, Christ died for us" (Romans 5:8).

I will never be able to overcome my patterns of sexual sin.

The Lie: Our sexual and emotional desires are out of our control. Those of us who experience same-sex attraction will never be free of what feels so natural to us. Those of us who compulsively have sex outside marriage are unable to control our urges and desires. Those who for years have self-soothed via masturbation will never be able to be free of this addiction. This is just how we are, and there's no point in trying to stop.

The Truth: It may feel this way at times, or even most of the time. However, to believe this is to say that Christ—and the power available to overcome sin through him—is insufficient. These struggles may last a long time, but that doesn't mean they *must* always win. Christ came to bring liberty to the captives (Luke 4:18); he *is* freeing us from our sins. To accept the lie that we cannot change is to give up in defeat. To believe that the possibility of change exists is to have the seed of hope necessary to fight against our sin. Cowards and heroes both fear death, but a coward gives up in defeat. A hero fights even unto death—and, to her surprise, wins!

My sin is worse and more abnormal than everyone else's sin.

The Lie: Women are to be proper and pure—which often can be translated as nonsexual. There's something seriously wrong with a woman who sins sexually. If she *enjoys* sinning sexually, she must be truly perverted. If she has sex with other women, she's clearly twisted. Nice women don't do these things.

The Truth: We often feel like lepers because of our sexual sin. We condemn ourselves, or believe the condemnation others have for us. It's true that people in the church tend to be shocked at sexual sin. Our measuring stick, however, is God's standard—that all sin originates and grows out of our wayward hearts (Matthew 15:18–19). The heart that manifests overeating, gossip, anger, and hatred is the same sinful heart that seeks to fulfill desires through sexual fantasy and behavior. Our hearts declare, "I want what I want the way I want it! I don't care what God says about it!" Sexual sin may have interpersonal consequences that other sins don't, but it is not a *worse* sin. Paul's remarks in 1 Corinthians 6:18–20 speak to the impact of sexual sin on other people, but are not to be seen as saying sexual sin is a *worse* sin than other sins.

Common lies about self and others:

This is just the way I am.

The Lie: Depending on the specific type of struggle we have, we say things like, "I was born gay. I need to embrace my same-sex desires, since I cannot change." Or, "I have always been more sexual than other women. That's how I was made. Call me an addict if you want, but there's no way for me *not* to give in to these desires."

The Truth: The Bible says we are all born with sinful hearts and natures (Romans 3:23, 5:12; Psalm 51:5). Yet, despite what we may hear, there is no conclusive evidence of a physiological, genetic *cause* of homosexuality The causes for same-sex attraction are complex and most likely have multiple and different pathways for each person. Simple reductionism ("I was born this way" or "it's just a choice") explains little and is ultimately unhelpful.

The particular type of sexual sin we pursue seems to be the result of our sinful heart (seed) interacting with and responding to the particular influences around us (soil). This doesn't mean we have an excuse to sin or that we cannot change and make different choices. Jesus told the woman caught in adultery to "go and sin no more" (John 8:11). This statement reveals that, through Christ's work in our lives and the enabling grace he gives, we can change the way we think and act, even if our inward temptations remain.

All men want one thing, and therefore can't be trusted.

The Lie: Men are controlled by sexual lust and only want woman for sex. Men will manipulate women to have sex with them and don't care what a woman is thinking or feeling. Men generally live out of a belief system that gives them permission to abuse and misuse vulnerable girls and women.

The Truth: Many women have had painful and detrimental experiences with men. Many of us have been abused as children and adolescents, and perhaps as adult women. The fact is men *are* sinful, but *so are women*. It's important to realize we are no better than men, and that we have sinned against them as well. Everyone is in need of a Savior and Redeemer who can change selfish desires, including sexual lusts. If we believe we can be saved and changed into Christlike women, we need to believe that men can also be changed by the Lord. Some of us have shown disdain and contempt for the male image of God through hatred of men. Others have sexually used and manipulated men in order to feel powerful and have a sense of control over them. Christ calls us to repent of selfish, unbiblical attitudes and seek to change our perspective, learning to view men as individuals rather than as a collective whole. While you might not be able to trust men in general, there may be particular godly men who God brings into your life. There are many men who love Jesus, respect women, and can be trusted.

All women are malicious gossips.

The Lie: Other women cannot be trusted. If we share anything, they will betray our trust.

The Truth: All women are sinners, yet this lie exaggerates the particular sin of some women and keeps us from having close friendships with others. It separates us from the world of women and says, "I am not going to be like *that.*" When we think this way, we reveal a haughty and prideful heart that looks down at other women and their sin issues. We cast stones at women whose besetting sins are "below" us in some way. How is this different from people doing that to *us* about *our* sexual sins?

I am not like other women; I'm "other" from them.

The Lie: We believe that, because of our sexual compulsions, attractions to women, or lack of attraction to men, we're different in our core identity as women. Our experience of being female feels radically different from what we hear other women express. Other women seem to deal with "normal" sins that Christians talk about more readily. They definitely don't talk about what *we* struggle with, so we must be abnormal sinners.

The Truth: For women who believe this lie, there is a sense of living outside the "world of women." We feel somehow abnormal and stuck in a neuter or male category. It keeps us from embracing our femininity and learning to experience the fullness of God's plan for us as women. God chose you to be a woman, with specific likes and dislikes, personality traits, physical characteristics, and even learning styles. The world is not the judge of what it means to be male or female. Defining masculinity and femininity must come from a biblical view of gender, not cultural views. Both male and female stereotypes have helped us feel like we don't fit in, and keep us from discovering and accepting who we are as women. Our true measure is Christ. We are to pursue how Christ specifically and uniquely made each of us. As we align our sense of identity and femininity to the word of God and through our relationship with Christ, we learn to embrace our womanhood.

I am more like a man than a woman because I...

The Lie: Perhaps because you happen to drive a pickup truck, like the color black, have short hair, are athletically inclined or built, enjoy tools, think logically and/or sequentially, and/or are visually stimulated, this means you're masculine. Or, if you pursue and enjoy sex (even heterosexually), you are more like a man than a woman because women do not aggressively pursue sex.

The Truth: You have gifts, talents, styles, and propensities that God has built and created within you. They are good qualities—and if you have them as a woman, then they *are* feminine. God is the maker and definer of what is feminine, not the stereotypes we hear. God chose you to be female, and he chose how you're made. You *are* female, no matter what the stereotypes of our culture say.

Men/women are inferior, and not as valuable as women/men.

The Lie: One gender is to be treasured over the other. Depending on where our cravings take us, we disdain what we don't crave and worship what we do.

The Truth: Our experiences and cravings may have us convinced that life and security is found in the gender that is the focus of our lusts. This lie is fueled by an attitude of pride and selfishness in our interpretations of others. But God created humanity male and female, and we are not to despise a portion of his creation. We're all created differently, uniquely, and equally sinful. We need to examine our hearts and see what attitudes we hold toward others.

Sex equals love.

The Lie: Some of us think that love and sex are the same. If we love someone, then we *will* have sex with that person. If someone loves us, that person *will* be sexual with us.

The Truth: This lie equates love and sex. Maybe the only time we've felt connected to someone is when we were being touched or talked to in a sexual way. Thus, we've learned to equate love with sexual touch and intercourse. But this is not how God reveals true love in the Bible. Love is shown by Jesus on the cross; love expresses itself in giving and sacrifice. Sexually using someone is not giving, nor is it sacrificial—it is taking and consuming for the satisfaction of selfish desires. Sex does not define a relationship, and having sex with someone does not prove love.

APPENDIX F
THE TWO TREES OF CODEPENDENCY

THE CODEPENDENT WHO SERVES

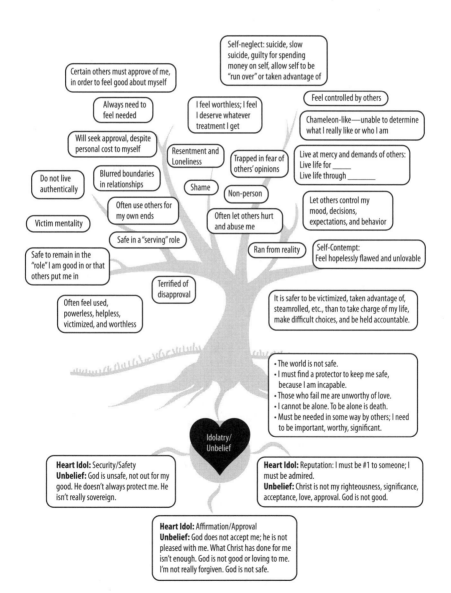

APPENDIX F *Continued*

THE CODEPENDENT WHO CONTROLS

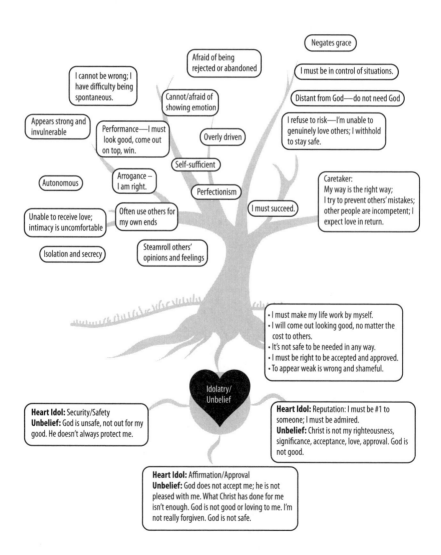

Negates grace

I must be in control of situations.

Afraid of being rejected or abandoned

Distant from God—do not need God

I cannot be wrong; I have difficulty being spontaneous.

Cannot/afraid of showing emotion

I refuse to risk—I'm unable to genuinely love others; I withhold to stay safe.

Appears strong and invulnerable

Performance—I must look good, come out on top, win.

Overly driven

Caretaker:
My way is the right way;
I try to prevent others' mistakes;
other people are incompetent; I expect love in return.

Self-sufficient

Autonomous

Arrogance – I am right.

Perfectionism

I must succeed.

Unable to receive love; intimacy is uncomfortable

Often use others for my own ends

Isolation and secrecy

Steamroll others' opinions and feelings

• I must make my life work by myself.
• I will come out looking good, no matter the cost to others.
• It's not safe to be needed in any way.
• I must be right to be accepted and approved.
• To appear weak is wrong and shameful.

Idolatry/ Unbelief

Heart Idol: Security/Safety
Unbelief: God is unsafe, not out for my good. He doesn't always protect me.

Heart Idol: Reputation: I must be #1 to someone; I must be admired.
Unbelief: Christ is not my righteousness, significance, acceptance, love, approval. God is not good.

Heart Idol: Affirmation/Approval
Unbelief: God does not accept me; he is not pleased with me. What Christ has done for me isn't enough. God is not good or loving to me. I'm not really forgiven. God is not safe.

ENDNOTES

Session 6
1. Lori Rentzel, *Emotional Dependency* (Downers Grove, IL: InterVarsity Press, 1990), 7.

Session 8
2. David Powlison, *Seeing with New Eyes: Counseling and the Human Condition Through the Lens of Scripture* (Phillipsburg, NJ: P&R Publishing, 2003).

Session 9
3. Dan Allender, *The Wounded Heart* (Colorado Springs, CO: NavPress, 1990), 48.
4. Allender, *The Wounded Heart Workbook* (Colorado Springs, CO: NavPress, 1992), 29.

Session 10
5. ESV Study Bible (Wheaton, IL: Crossway Bibles, 2008), 2273.
6. Thomas à Kempis, *Of the Imitation of Christ* (New Kensington, PA: Whitaker House, 1981), 135.

Session 13
7. Elyse Fitzpatrick, *Idols of the Heart: Learning to Long for God Alone* (Phillipsburg, NJ: P&R Publishing, 2001), 23.
8. Ibid., 64–65.

Session 14
9. Chris Thurman, *The Lies We Believe* (Nashville, TN: Thomas Nelson Publishers, 1999), 5-6.

Session 16
10. Patrick Carnes, *Out of the Shadows* (Center City, MN: Hazelden Publishing, 2001), 26.

Session 17
11. Dave White, "Temptation as Suffering," Harvest USA Newsletter (Fall/Winter 2008). Available at www.harvestusa.org.

12. Lysa TerKeurst, *Made to Crave: Satisfying Your Deepest Desire With God, Not Food* (Grand Rapids, MI: Zondervan, 2010).

Session 19
13. Much of the information contained in this section is taken from the article, "Close Friends or Entangled Hearts?" by Ellen Dykas, *The Journal of Biblical Counseling*, Winter 2006 Volume 24, Number 1.

Appendix A
14. Dan Wilson, PhD, "God Gives the Best Sex: A Positive Theology of Sex," Harvest USA Newsletter (Fall 2007). Available at www.harvestusa.org.

Appendix D
15. Sarah Lipp, "Anger and Sex: A Woman's Perspective from the Trenches," *Harvest News*, (Winter 2006). Available at www.harvestusa.org.

Resources for Further Study:
Session 9: The Soil: Traumatic Pain
- Dan Allender, *The Wounded Heart* (Colorado Springs, CO: NavPress, 1990).
- Kay Arthur, *Lord, Heal My Hurts* (Colorado Springs, CO: Waterbrook Press, 2000).
- Diane Langberg, *On the Threshold of Hope* (Carol Stream, IL: Tyndale House Publishers, 1999).
- Dan McCartney, *Why Does It Have to Hurt?* (Phillipsburg, NJ: P & R Publishing Company, 1997).

- Joni Eareckson Tada and Steve Estes, *When God Weeps* (Grand Rapids, MI: Zondervan Publishing House, 1997).

Session 11: Looking for Your Emotional Home in All the Wrong Places

- Ellen Dykas, *When Women's Friendships Turn Sexual: Finding Our Home in Jesus.* Harvest USA Newsletter (Fall 2010). Available at www.harvestusa.org.
- David Powlison, "Peace Be Still: Psalm 131," chapter in *Seeing with New Eyes: Counseling and the Human Condition Through the Lens of Scripture* (Phillipsburg, NJ: P&R Publishing, 2003).

Appendix C: Thoughts on Parent-Child Bonding

- Tim Clinton and Gary Sibcy, *Attachments: Why You Love, Feel, and ACT the Way You Do* (Nashville, TN: Thomas Nelson Publishers, 2002).
- Henry Cloud and John Townsend, *The Mom Factor* (Grand Rapids, MI: Zondervan, 1996).
- Janelle Hallman, *The Heart of Female Same-sex Attraction: A Comprehensive Counseling Resource* (Downers Grove, IL: InterVarsity Press, 2008).
- Brenda Hunter, *In the Company of Women* (Sisters, OR: Multnomah Books, 1994).
- David Stoop, *Making Peace with Your Father* (Ventura, CA: Regal Books, 2004).
- Winston Smith, Book Review of *The Practice of Emotionally Focused Couple Therapy:*
- *Creating Connection* (The Journal of Biblical Counseling, Volume 26 No. 1).

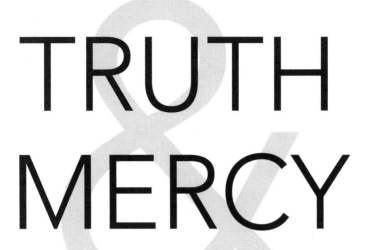

TRUTH & MERCY

Harvest USA brings the truth and mercy of Jesus Christ to men, women, and families affected by sexual sin and equips the church to minister to sexually broken people. We are a faith-operated, missions ministry. Most of our work is given freely or at low cost. We are primarily supported by churches and individuals convinced of our mission.

If you have found this book helpful, consider partnering with us by giving financially, advocating for our ministry in your church, and/or by volunteering your time. For questions, counsel, and opportunities to help, please contact:

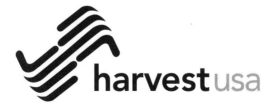

3901B Main Street, Suite 304
Philadelphia, PA 19127
215.482.0111
info@harvestusa.org
www.harvestusa.org

For Harvest USA resources visit **www.harvest-usa-store.com**
or call 336.378.7775